Shrewd Food

Shrewd Food

60 Ways to Eat Yourself Healthy

NOONIE ZAND GOODARZI

ILLUSTRATIONS BY MUDD BEXLEY

Publisher: Badger Books Ltd, 2024

All rights reserved. No part of this publication may be reproduced, distributed, or transmitted in any form or by any means, including photocopying, recording, or other electronic or mechanical methods, without the prior written permission of the copyright holder and the publisher, except in the case of brief quotations embodied in critical reviews and certain other non-commercial uses permitted by copyright law.

The moral right of Noonie Zand Goodarzi to be identified as the author and compiler of this work has been asserted.

© Noonie Zand Goodarzi, 2024

978-1-0685854-0-1 –Print
978-1-0685854-1-8 - eBook

Insta: @izustrations

Cover and interior illustrations by Mudd Bexley.

Book design by Principal Publishing.

Publisher website: nialledworthy.com

Email: niall@nialledworthy.com

Insta: @nialledworthybooks

For Babak, Violet & Edie

Contents

Foreword xi

Match your calorie intake to the path of the sun 1
Eat smaller portions and chew your food well 3
Start each meal with vegetables and protein 5
Avoid naked carbs.. 7
Seek out quercetin 9
Get with the beets 11
Make a friend of broccoli... 13
Limit exposure to free radicals 15
Eat up your greens... 17
Sprinkle on some flaxseeds.. 19
Drink green tea and relax.. 21
Don't shrink away from garlic....................................... 23
Feast on fermented foods... 25
Beware of added sugar 27
A smoothie a day (but hold the banana)....................... 29
Don't get thirsty 31
Feel free to go nuts.. 33
Raise your pulse rate 35
Think bitters for bile flow... 37
Go to work on an egg.. 39
Feel the magic of mushrooming 41
Get your kicks from chocolate 43
Be generous with the olive oil....................................... 45

Reap the benefits of berries *47*
Eat before alcohol *49*
Watch your cravings *51*
Fill up on fibre *53*
Avoid nasty chemicals *55*
Have a little fishy on a little dishy *57*
An apple a day *59*
Go wild in the country *61*
Get sprouting *63*
Put out inflammatory fire with turmeric *65*
Think twice about processed meats *67*
Appreciate the genius of ginger *69*
Shake the salt habit *71*
Be wholeheartedly whole grain *73*
Think herbs and spice and all things nice *75*
Go pear-shaped *77*
Embrace female-friendly phytoestrogens *79*
Eat yourself happy *81*
Wake up and smell the coffee *83*
Get well on bone broth *85*
Use pumpkin seeds for prostate health *87*
Go guacamole *89*
Take a stroll after eating *91*
Get creative with salads *93*
Lower your blood pressure with hibiscus tea ... *95*
Sort out your fats *97*
Indulge in a little of what you fancy *99*
Use adaptogens for stress management *101*

Add in some raw food *103*
Feed your thyroid *105*
Remember variety is the spice of life *107*
Get rootsy *109*
Know your non-dairy milks.. *111*
Choose the right cinnamon.. *113*
Balance your protein... *115*
To snack or not to snack? *117*
Get a better night's sleep.. *119*

Acknowledgements *121*
About the Author *123*

Foreword

As the early Greek physician Hippocrates advised, we should make food our medicine. We all want to live long and healthy lives and the food that we eat is probably the most important determinant of the metabolic programming of our cells.

Unlike stress and pollution, our diet is something that is actively within our control and a lovely study in the *Journal of the American College of Cardiology* brought home to me how our dietary choices really do matter.

In the study, researchers looked at the immediate effect that food has on certain health markers, including inflammation, excess free radicals, and high blood glucose, and they found that damage to our arteries occurs after just one unhealthy meal (cheeseburger, chips, fizzy drink).

The study then goes on to say that our bodies begin to repair that damage by "exerting profound and immediate favourable changes" following just one healthy meal (salmon, salad, green tea).

These results are an inspiring reminder of the medicinal power of food - of how responsive we are to the things that we eat, and of how our actions have consequences, hopefully positive.

I have written this book, then, as a means of offering a series of simple, but life-changing nutritional tips that are easy to implement and will benefit your health enormously if you put them into action.

Try and achieve even one a day and you'll slowly start to reap the rewards.

Noonie Zand Goodarzi

"What most people don't realise is that food is not just calories; it's information. It actually contains messages that connect to every cell in the body"
Dr. Mark Hyman

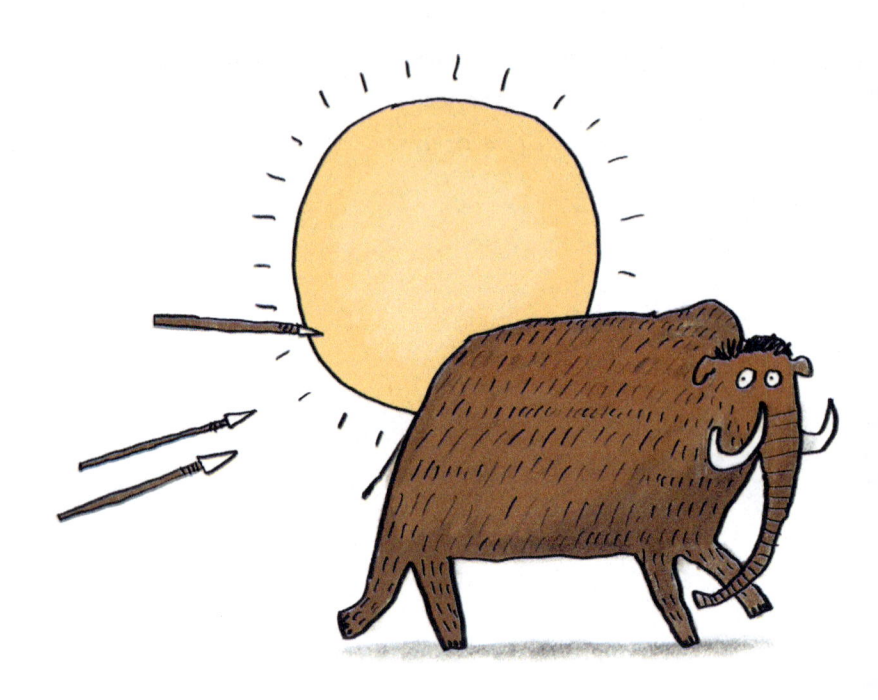

Match your calorie intake to the path of the sun

Due to our circadian rhythm, or internal body clock, our ability to handle glucose diminishes as the day progresses and the light ebbs. Pre-fire, our ancestors would rise and sleep with the sun and were not programmed to eat under cover of darkness. As a result of this ancient biology, trials have shown that eating at 8pm can cause double the blood sugar response from the identical meal eaten at 8am.

Late lunches aren't great either – people who eat a large lunch at 4.30pm can have a 46 per cent bigger blood sugar spike than those who eat the same at 1pm. Tucking into food after 11pm can also disrupt the metabolism for hours, causing significantly higher blood sugar after breakfast the next day. In short, frequently raised blood glucose is not a good thing. Glucose is toxic to our cells and tissues, plus it means higher levels of insulin, which is very ageing.

So, eat your largest meals before 1pm and avoid sugar and refined carbs at night when your body is not well equipped to deal with them. It will improve your sleep too.

Did you know?... Remains found in a cave in South Africa show that campfires were burning as long as a million years ago. The discovery of fire enabled our ancestors to keep warm, cook food, fend off animals, travel into colder areas and, crucially, to stay together in groups – and it was this that promoted the development of language.

2   Noonie Zand Goodarzi

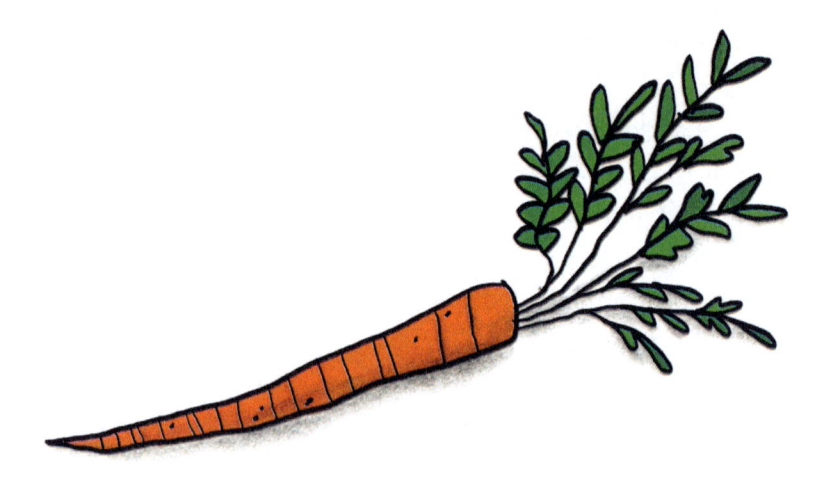

Eat smaller portions and chew your food well

Chewing food well is a key part of the digestive process. Food needs to be broken down into liquid before it reaches our stomach for digestive enzymes to work optimally.

It has been shown that if you consciously take time with your food and chew properly, you won't eat as much, and therefore your body won't have to produce so much insulin, a hormone that causes excess blood glucose to be turned into fat. After 20 minutes your brain will register that your stomach is full, so try to delay going up for a second helping – you'll find you won't need it.

A good exercise is to stop and take several deep breaths into your belly whenever you sit down for a meal. This will relax you by stimulating your parasympathetic nervous system and make you more mindful of what you are eating. Savour that first (best) mouthful and stop eating before you are full.

> **Did you know?...** Digestion starts in the mouth with the enzyme amylase in our saliva. An adult human produces about 1-2 litres of saliva every day from salivary glands. This is about 23,000 litres of saliva during an average lifetime. That's a whole lot of spit!

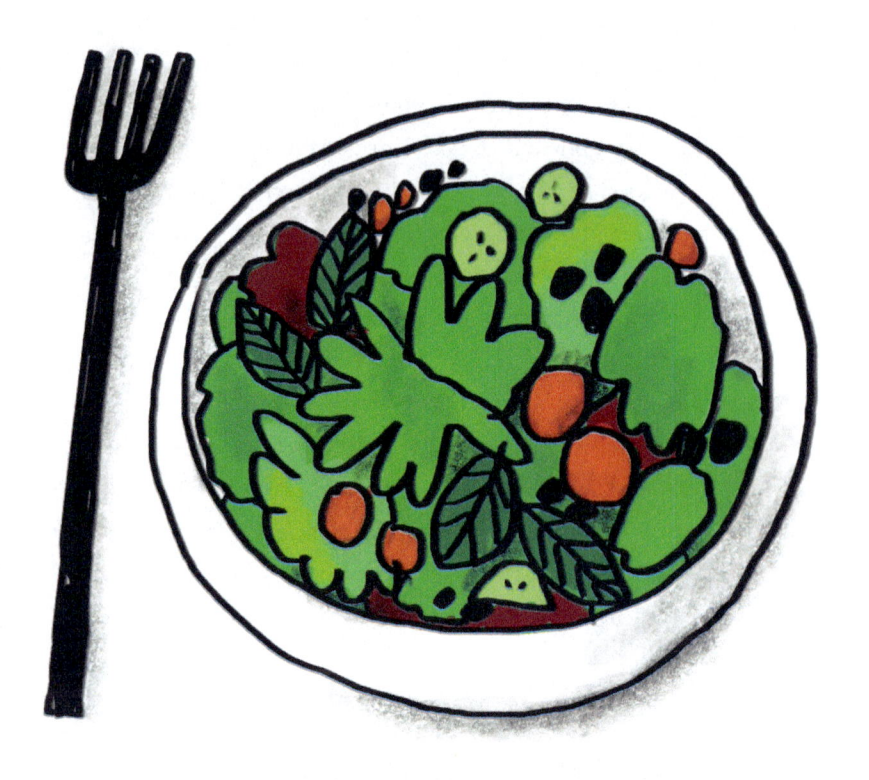

Start each meal with vegetables and protein

Studies have shown that the way we sequence foods matters. If we eat vegetables at the beginning of a meal containing carbohydrates like rice, pasta or bread, the fibre forms a gel-like substance in the gut which prevents our blood sugar from spiking after the carbs.

Similarly, foods that are higher in fat and protein take longer to digest because the food stays in the stomach for longer. So, if you are eating a carb-heavy meal, think about starting with a mixed salad with an olive oil dressing – and always eat the vegetables and protein on your plate first.

Researchers in Japan found that eating meat or fish and vegetables before white rice not only helps the body to prevent high blood sugar but also to secrete a hormone which makes you feel full. Another option is to 'pre-load' on a handful of almonds. One study showed that 12 almonds before a heavy meal improved blood sugar responses for pre-diabetic people; in another, body fat was significantly lowered after 16 weeks, including dangerous visceral fat.

> **Did you know?...** While most people know them as nuts, almonds are actually classified as drupes – a type of fruit that is fleshy on the outside with a shell covering a seed on the inside. The almond is the seed.

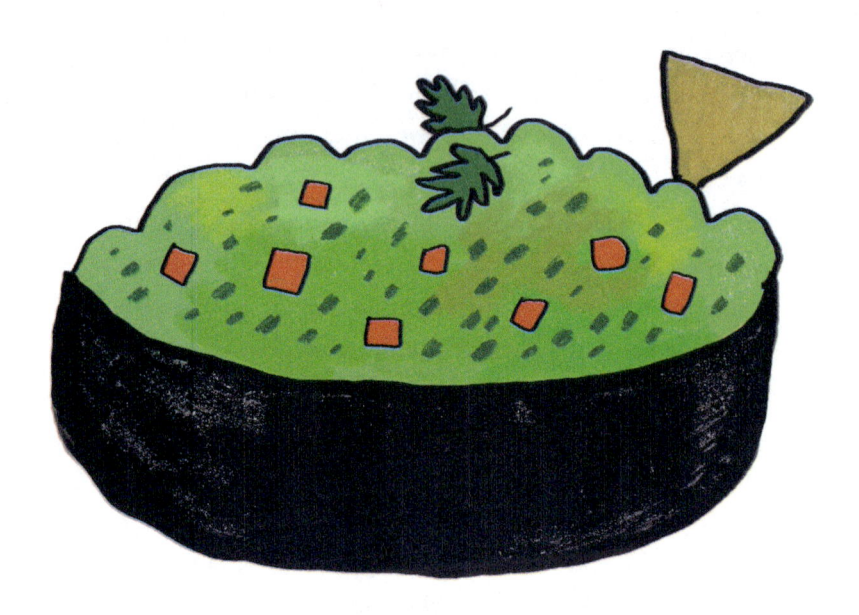

Avoid naked carbs

Resist eating carbs on their own – that is, without protein, fat or fibre. Keeping blood sugar levels balanced is an important aspect of ageing well and recent research links high insulin to many of the age-related diseases including diabetes, heart disease, cancer and Alzheimer's.

When you have a piece of toast and jam, a bowl of packet cereal or a handful of tortilla chips, these refined carbs quickly get broken down into glucose in the bloodstream which then triggers the body to release insulin. Too much insulin, like glucose, is damaging to our cells and tissues: it causes DNA to turn over more quickly; triggers inflammation; damages antioxidant stores; and raises levels of bad LDL cholesterol. All in all, not a great CV.

Choose high-fibre, wholemeal versions of wheat and rice, and if you are going to have a carb snack, make sure that you pair it with some protein, fibre and healthy fats – a piece of toast with nut butter; tortilla chips with guacamole; a handful of nuts and seeds with cereal. This will slow down the rate that the carbs are digested and reduce the dreaded glucose spike.

Did you know?... The deadliest combination for blood sugar is to have your carbohydrate snack with a coffee. Those in a study who had a coffee-carb combo had triple the increase in blood sugar levels. Something to think about the next time you step into Starbucks and eye up that croissant.

Noonie Zand Goodarzi

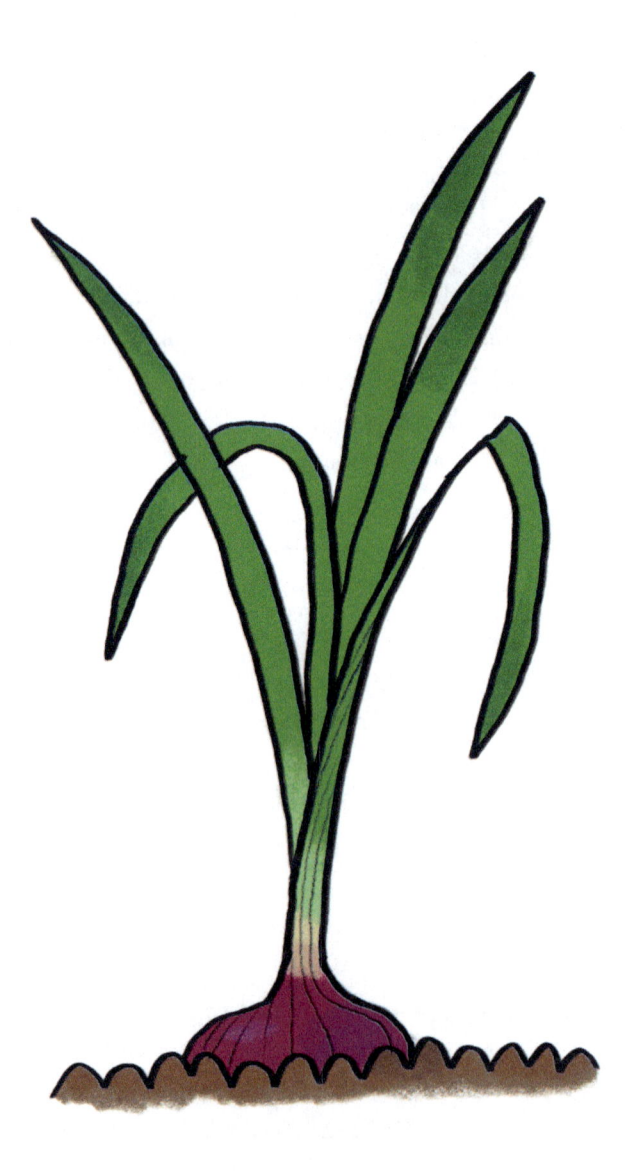

Seek out quercetin

Quercetin is a plant chemical called a flavonoid, and it is a particularly punchy one. Known for its anti-inflammatory, antioxidant and anti-allergy properties, quercetin has been shown to mediate inflammation caused by nasty chemicals in the body called free radicals.

It also has positive effects on high blood pressure, high uric acid levels in gout, pain and stiffness in rheumatoid arthritis, as well as being great for people with allergies as it prevents cells from releasing histamine. For all these reasons, it is a no-brainer to include more of it in your diet.

High amounts of quercetin are found in capers, red onions, apples with their skins, and dark chocolate; smaller amounts are in coriander, kale, dill, sorrel, red grapes, black and green tea, cherries and citrus fruit (particularly the zest).

Make a point of including foods that contain quercetin every day – a bit of raw red onion and coriander in a salad, a few capers in a tomato sauce, some dill and lemon zest on grilled fish. Whatever it is, find ways to add it in.

Did you know?... Red onions are a notable source of quercetin, but don't let them sit around in the cupboard for long. If you can get an onion fresh from the ground, all the better, as onions lose up to 33 percent of their quercetin after just 12 days of storage.

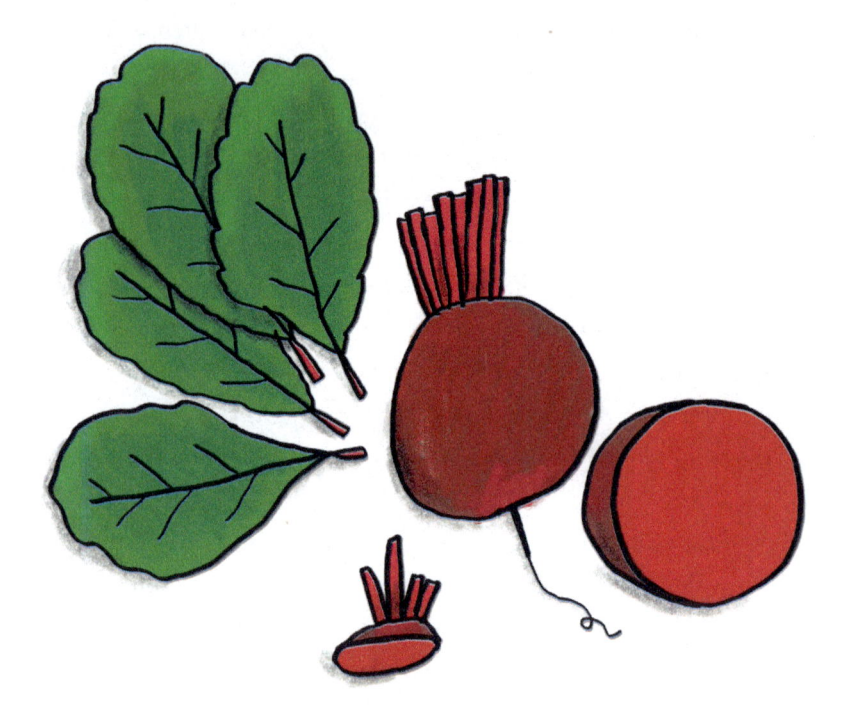

Get with the beets

Beetroot deserves a special mention because it is such a powerhouse of a root. It is packed with nutrients, contains an antioxidant and anti-inflammatory red pigment, plus it helps our cells work more efficiently due to its high nitrate content.

When eaten, nitrates are transformed into nitric oxide which dilates the coronary arteries allowing more oxygenated blood to flow to the heart, lowering blood pressure. Beets are also full of vitamins A & C, folate, potassium, iron, and manganese, plus the antioxidant betalain, that not only protects against damaging oxidative stress, but also helps to support liver detoxification processes.

In short, beetroot is nothing short of a superfood superstar. No excuse not to try them because they are cheap and deliciously versatile – eat them raw in a salad, steamed, boiled, roasted, pickled, juiced or even added to chocolate cake. Don't make the mistake of throwing away the green tops as they are equally nutritious. Steam them with the beets and serve like the Greeks do with lots of olive oil.

> **Did you know?...** In 1975, when the Cold War was easing between America and the USSR, the rival astronaut crews joined vessels in space and exchanged a famous handshake. As a goodwill gesture, the Russians handed over tubes of what looked like vodka, but which were in fact borscht, a hearty beetroot soup.

Noonie Zand Goodarzi

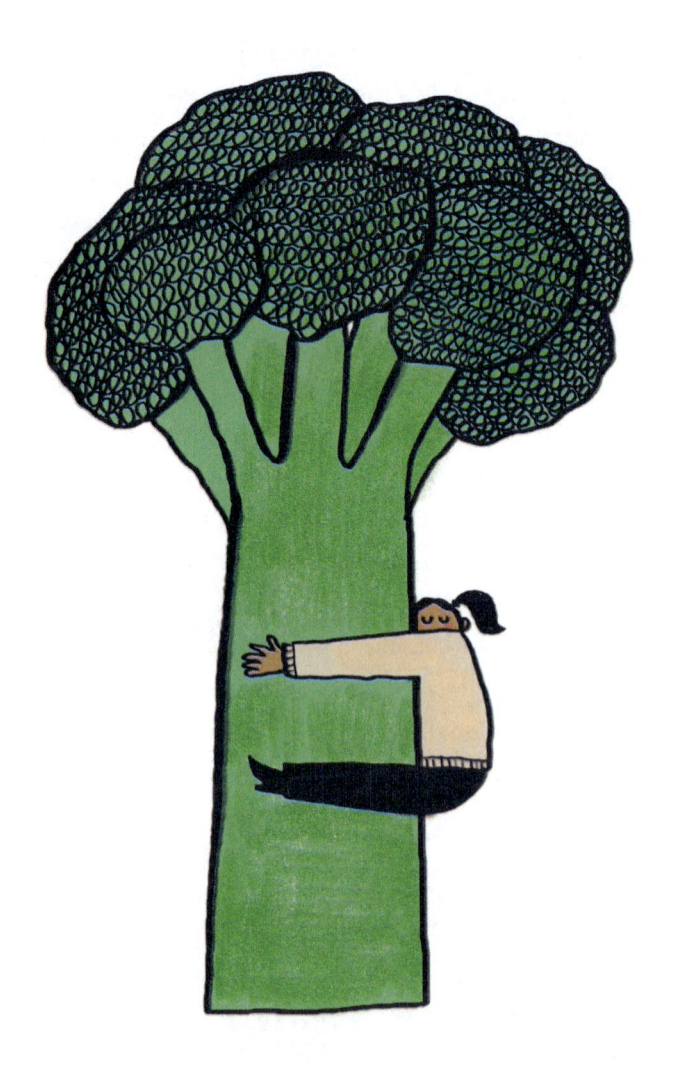

Make a friend of broccoli

Broccoli is part of the cruciferous vegetable clan known as 'The Brassicas' and, such is their power, it is nutritionally wise to make them your friend. Brassicas include rocket, bok choy, Brussels sprouts, cabbage, cauliflower, horseradish, kale, kohlrabi, radishes, watercress and broccoli – and their potency comes from a miraculous compound called sulforaphane.

Studies have shown that sulforaphane can prevent DNA damage from smoking; stop metastatic cancer spread; boost liver detox enzymes; and protect cells from pollutants. One mistake that people make is to boil their brassicas, thus inactivating the sulforaphane. Instead, chop and leave for forty minutes before cooking, which preserves the goodness, and be aware that frozen veg lack sulforaphane as they are flash-boiled before going into the freezer.

Have a daily serving of cruciferous vegetables and get creative in finding ways to add them in – horseradish to mashed potato; kale crisps; garnishes of red cabbage or rocket; a crunchy radish snack; home-sprouted broccoli sprouts. Your body will thank you.

> **Did you know?...** People who hate Brussels sprouts have a particular gene that makes them perceive bitterness in certain foods. It appears that boiling the veg is the worst taste-wise, but roasting them helps mask the bitterness – or combining with garlic, balsamic vinegar, or lemon juice.

14 Noonie Zand Goodarzi

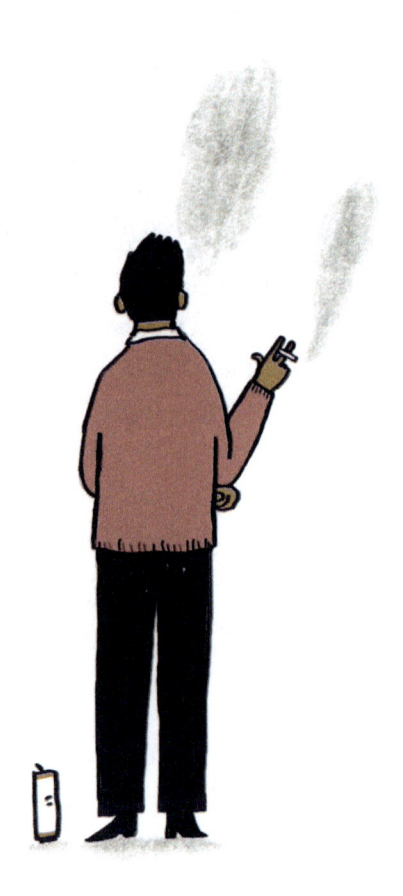

Limit exposure to free radicals

Oxidative stress and inflammation are two processes that go hand in hand when we age.

Free radicals or oxidants are produced by our bodies when our cells use oxygen to create energy, and a certain amount of them are used to good purpose in the body. However, they are also caused by a host of other more unfavourable things ranging from pollution to processed food and stress, and there is a danger that if they are left unchecked, they become rogue molecules that rampage around the body a bit like rust, causing damage to the DNA in our cells.

It is therefore crucial to make an effort to limit exposure to them. To put it simply, the worst thing you could do is to stand by the side of a busy polluted road on your mobile phone in the hot sun, letting your skin burn, breathing in the cars' fumes while eating some Pringles, smoking a fag and drinking a beer.

If you want to protect your body (particularly your heart and brain) from nasty, damaging molecules, don't do any of the above. Plus, it goes without saying, fill your diet with protective antioxidants.

Did you know?... In a long legal battle, Procter & Gamble claimed that Pringles were not crisps, but instead 'savoury snacks' as they contain only 42% potato flour. This was due to the UK tax on potato products that P&G didn't want to pay. Despite this unappetising claim, they were deemed crisps in 2009.

Noonie Zand Goodarzi

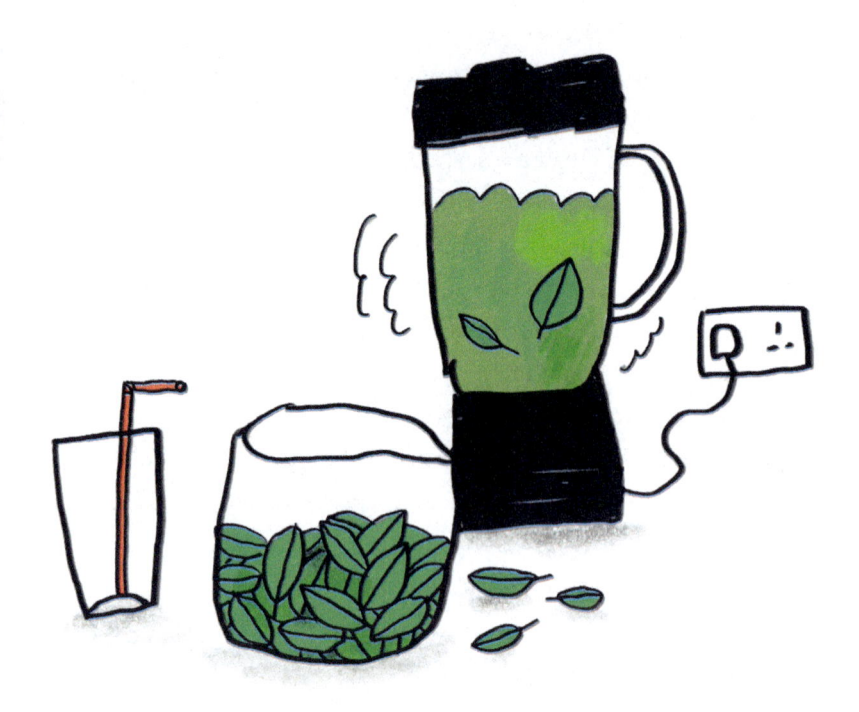

Eat up your greens

Eating a daily portion of dark green leafy vegetables like spinach, Swiss chard, collard greens, kale or Cavolo Nero is one of the simplest but most powerful things you could do for your health.

Greens are amongst the healthiest foods out there. In a Harvard trial, they showed the strongest inverse association with major chronic disease of all the fruit and veg tested. Apart from their fibre, they are packed with Vitamins C, K, folate, beta-carotene, magnesium, iron, calcium, plus antioxidants called carotenoids. These powerful compounds are fat-soluble, so pair your greens with healthy fats like nuts, seeds, avocado or olive oil – it can triple the amount of nutrients that make it into your bloodstream.

The Greeks serve their *horta* – wild mountain greens – steamed, with olive oil and a wedge of lemon. Perfection on a plate! Add greens into as many meals as possible – some spinach in a smoothie; steamed kale with an egg; chard in a bean stew; or collard greens as a base for meat or fish.

> **Did you know?...** On a primitive psychological level, green is the colour that instils a feeling of peace and we are drawn towards it because our instinct tells us that where there is green, there is life. Another reason it feels so harmonious is that green lies in the middle of the light spectrum and our eyes require no adjustment to see it.

Noonie Zand Goodarzi

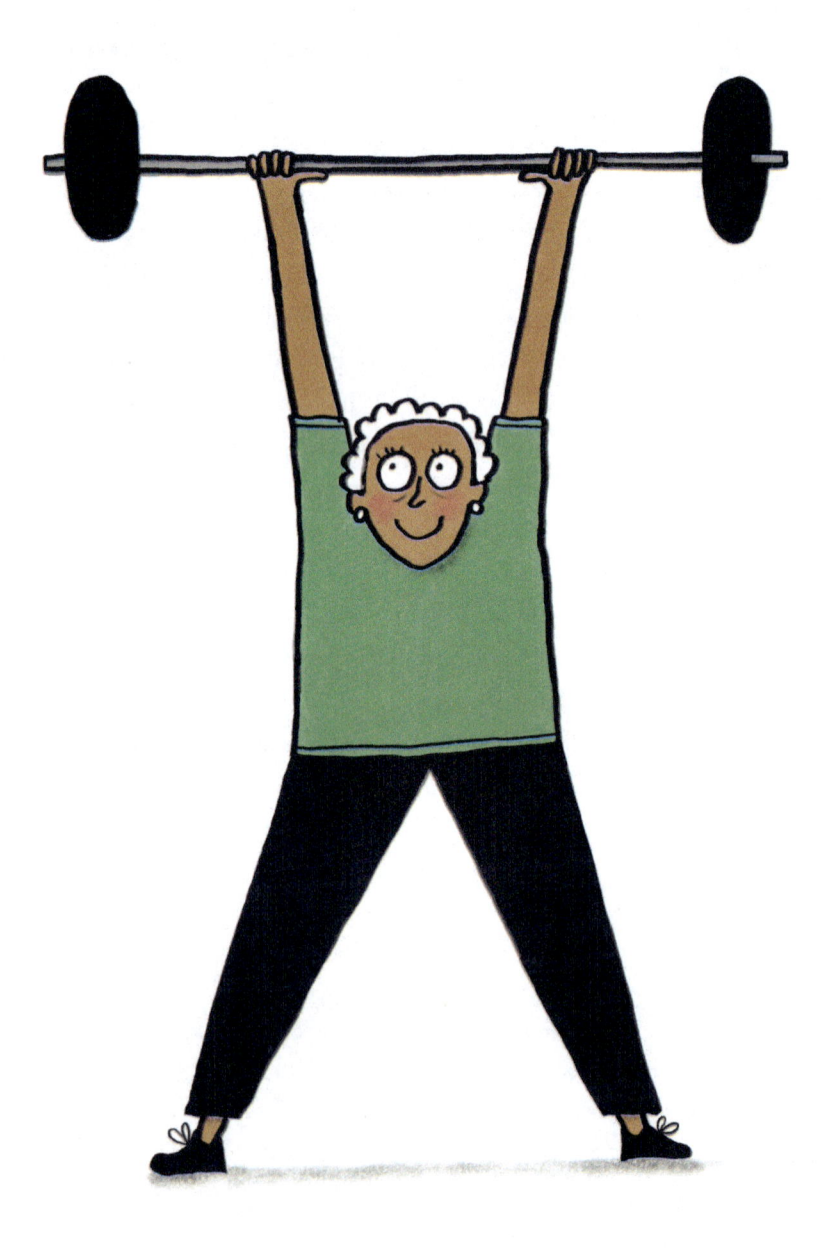

Sprinkle on some flaxseeds

These miraculous little seeds have been grown since the beginning of civilisation, and it's easy to see why. Also called linseeds, flaxseeds are a valuable plant source of anti-inflammatory omega-3 fat alpha-linoleic acid, plus they contain high amounts of phytoestrogens known as lignans.

These natural plant hormones help to create hormonal balance and trials have shown they can ease menopausal symptoms, plus reduce breast cancer growth and prostate cancer progression. Flaxseeds' high fibre content aids the removal of toxins out through the bowels, and studies have shown them useful for high blood pressure (working 2-3 times better than medical drugs), high cholesterol, and high blood sugar.

Be sure to grind the seeds, otherwise they pass through the gut with no benefit, and keep them refrigerated to stop the delicate fats from going rancid. Have 1-2 tablespoons per day and add to smoothies, cereal, yoghurt or porridge to deliver valuable breakfast protein. Also, use their oil in salad dressings or on steamed veg, but don't cook with it as it should not be heated.

> **Did you know?...** Hippocrates – the father of modern medicine – was big on flax for the relief of abdominal problems. Still today, flax is a tried and tested formula for constipation. Soak 4 teaspoons of flaxseeds in a third of a glass of water overnight, then add a teaspoon of the swollen seeds to food, or drink twice a day until you're regular.

Noonie Zand Goodarzi

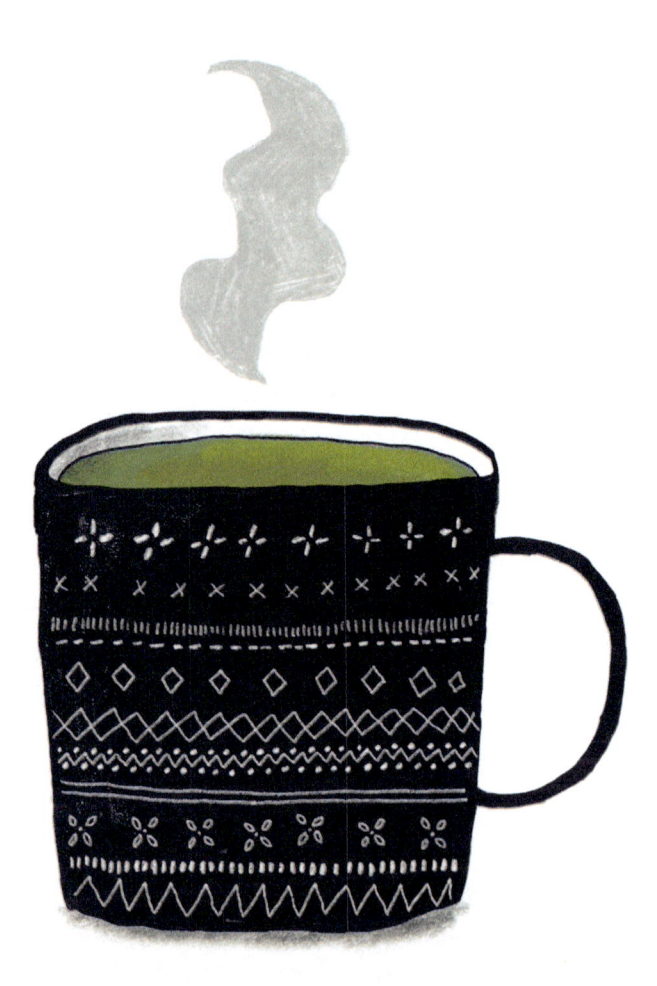

Drink green tea and relax

My friend who has meditated every day for thirty years has tried to explain the mental state one is aiming for in meditation: "You need to be as alert as a scientist and as relaxed as a hippy".

It struck me that what he was explaining was a bit like the effects of the amino acid L-theanine, which reduces anxiety and increases concentration at the same time – the holy grail of sensation. L-theanine is found almost solely in tea plants, particularly green tea like Gyokuro and Matcha, and drinking it can help you relax.

Other positives of green tea include its high antioxidant levels and liver protective properties. Four cups a day will deliver benefits, so if you find yourself mindlessly drinking coffee or black tea, think green. Matcha has 10 times more antioxidants than normal green tea so one cup goes a long way.

Avoid using boiling water in green tea as it releases the bitter tannins (80°C is ideal) and use plant-based milk in a matcha latte as cow's milk limits the bioavailability of the polyphenols.

> **Did you know?...** Green tea delivers quite a hit of caffeine too, with a typical cup containing 25-45 mg of caffeine – less than black tea, which is around 45-75 mg per cup. Coffee delivers between 95-200 mg per cup, while matcha green tea has 60-70 mg.

Noonie Zand Goodarzi

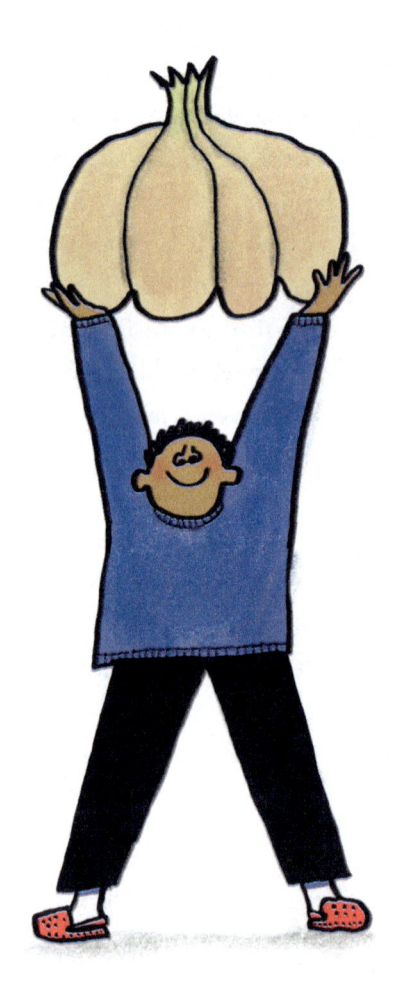

Don't shrink away from garlic

Sanskrit records show that garlic has been used remedially for over 5,000 years. It is no coincidence that in all the 'Blue Zones', known for the longevity of their inhabitants, garlic is not just an ingredient – it is the defining component of the diet.

This remarkable bulb contains the sulphur compound allicin to which most of its health benefits are attributed. Allicin is anti-cancer, antibacterial, anti-fungal, antiviral, anti-inflammatory, anti-diabetic, anti-hypertensive, cardio-protective and nephroprotective – need I go on? I mean, is there nothing this plant cannot do?

Add garlic to anything you cook in olive oil – also to soups, stews and sauces. Use raw in salad dressings and steamed vegetables, and chuck in whole bulbs when roasting meat.

To super-boost its healing properties, crush it rather than slice it as the more you damage garlic, the more allicin it releases. If possible, leave it to sit for 10-15 minutes before cooking as it will keep on releasing it.

Did you know?... In Funk & Wagnalls *Standard Dictionary of Folklore, Mythology, and Legend*, we are told that it is garlic's pungent smell that is responsible for the age-old belief of its power to drive away ghouls. Chew on fresh mint leaves to neutralise the whiff as they lower the concentration of smelly sulphur compounds.

24 Noonie Zand Goodarzi

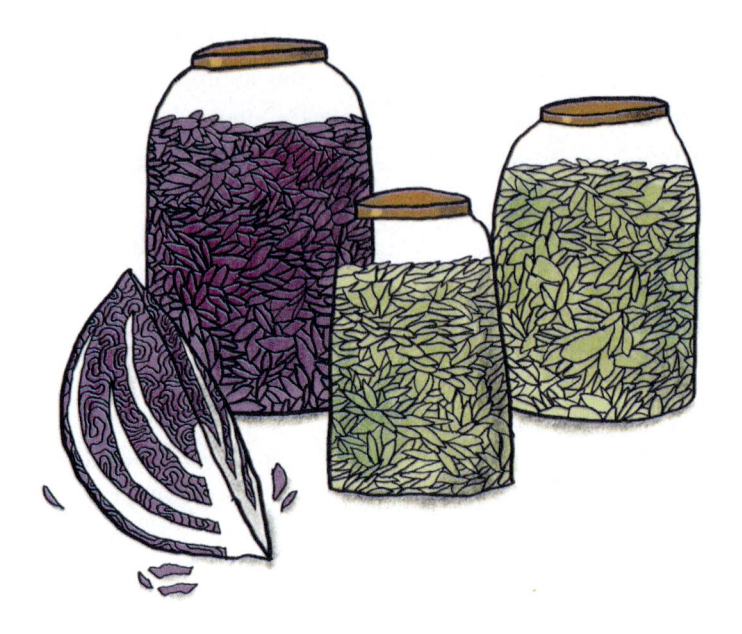

Feast on fermented foods

Good physical and mental health always starts with the gut.

Around 70-80% of our immune tissue is found within the digestive tract, alongside trillions of bacteria known as the microbiome. These gut bacteria play a vital role: they are potent detoxifiers, plus they significantly enhance the effectiveness of these local mucosal immune cells, as well as strengthening immunity in general. What is more, the microbiome is in constant communication with the brain via the vagus nerve and has been shown to exert significant benefits on mental health. It's all rather miraculous.

Maintaining a healthy balance of good gut bacteria is therefore vital, and an easy way we can do this is by eating fermented foods which naturally contain these live microorganisms. Have at least one portion daily – miso soup; raw apple cider vinegar in salad dressing; kimchi or sauerkraut as a relish; probiotic yoghurt for pudding; a glass of kefir at breakfast; or kombucha instead of alcohol. Try making sauerkraut or kombucha yourself – it's a lot easier than you think and extremely satisfying.

> **Did you know?...** The 100 trillion microbes of the microbiome are defined as all the bacteria, viruses, fungi, archaea, and eukaryotes that inhabit the human gut. It makes up over half the cells in the human body, weighs around 2 lbs, and is now considered a separate organ with its own distinct metabolic and immune activity.

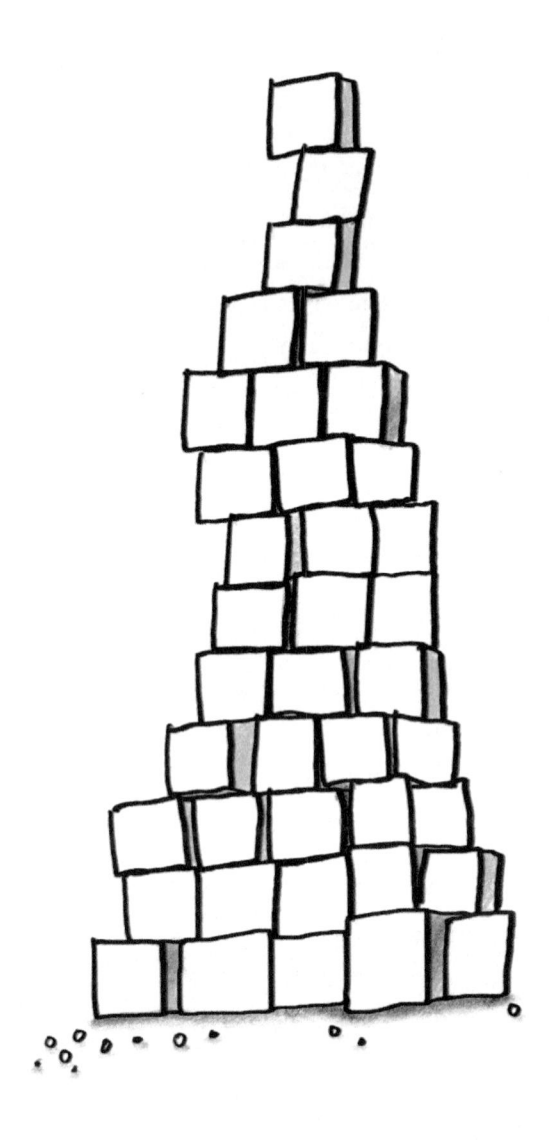

Beware of added sugar

We all know about sugar's impact on obesity and type 2 diabetes, but other pernicious effects abound: sugar triggers inflammation; disarms the immune system for several hours; disrupts the microbiome; raises blood pressure; reduces cognitive function; and can lead to fatty liver disease.

We get natural sugars in fruit and veg, but these are balanced by their fibre, so it is added sugars, as well as the sugars from refined carbs, that we need to watch. We are advised from 11 years old to eat no more than 30 grams, or 7 teaspoons, of (free) sugar a day – something surprisingly difficult unless you cook with fresh ingredients.

Food manufacturers like to sneak sugar into ready-made foods to encourage consumers to eat more. Look for hidden sugars like fructose, galactose, maltose, maltodextrin, brown rice syrup, corn syrup or barley malt in ingredient lists, and choose foods with no more than 5 grams of sugar per 100 grams. Also, watch out for foods that appear healthy, but are actually sugar-laden – low-fat yoghurts, fruit juice, pasta sauce, granola, ready oats, protein bars, sliced bread and honey. Best of all, cook from scratch so you know where you stand.

> **Did you know?**...One can of Coke contains 9 teaspoons of sugar; one glass of orange juice – 5–6 tsps; one dollop of tomato ketchup – 1 tsp; 1 dollop sweet chilli sauce – 2 tsps; low fat fruit yoghurt – 4-7 tsps; a helping of granola – 2.5 tsps; slice of white bread – 0.5 tsps; 1 glass of dry white wine around 0.25 tsps.

Noonie Zand Goodarzi

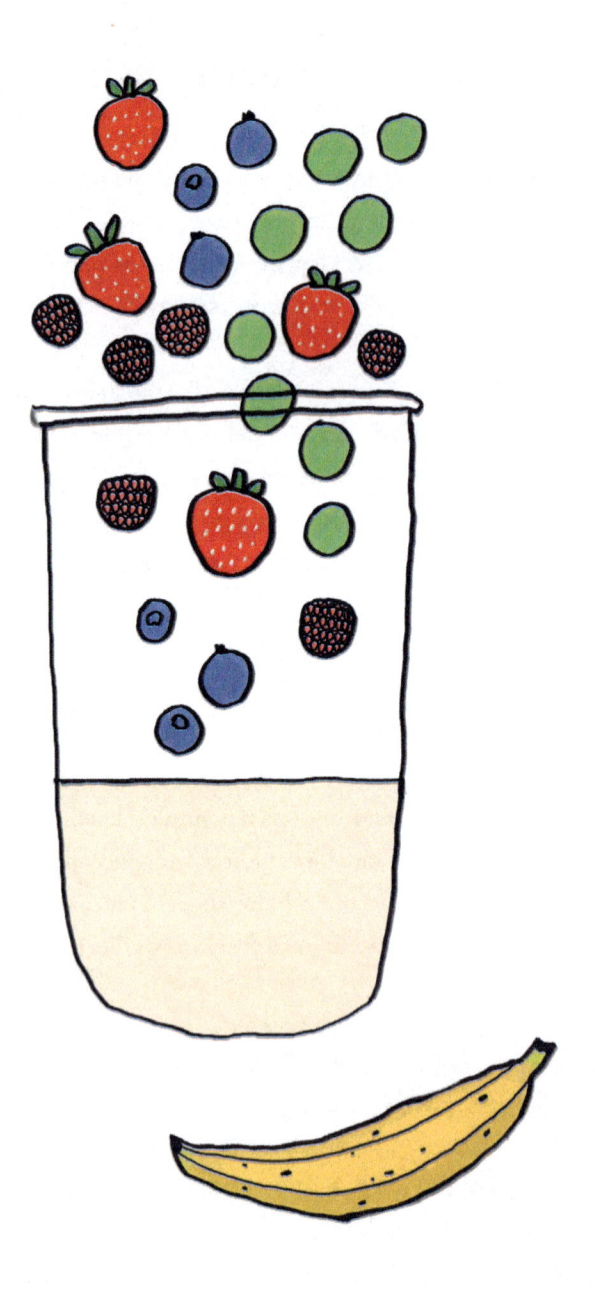

A smoothie a day (but hold the banana)

Berries and bananas have always jumped happily hand in hand into a smoothie, but annoyingly a new study has shown that an enzyme in bananas actually decreases the bioavailability of the flavanol antioxidants in berries by a whopping 84%.

Flavanols are found in high amounts in apples, pears, berries, grapes and cocoa, and studies have shown that they improve the circulation of oxygen around the body, notably benefitting the heart, brain and skin. To gain their full healing power, avoid blending them with banana. Use alternatives such as avocado, probiotic Greek yoghurt, or even a small amount of pre-steamed cauliflower, which will give you a similar creamy texture.

A smoothie for breakfast needs added protein to stop it from spiking your blood sugar: a tablespoon of ground flaxseed; 2 teaspoons of nut butter; a good quality protein powder; half an avocado; some pre-soaked chia seeds; a cup of probiotic yoghurt; or a combination of the above. This will help to keep you going until lunchtime.

> **Did you know?**...The banana is actually scientifically a berry, whereas the strawberry is not. The strict classification of a berry is that it must contain seeds inside the flesh, like a banana, rather than on the outside, like a strawberry.

Noonie Zand Goodarzi

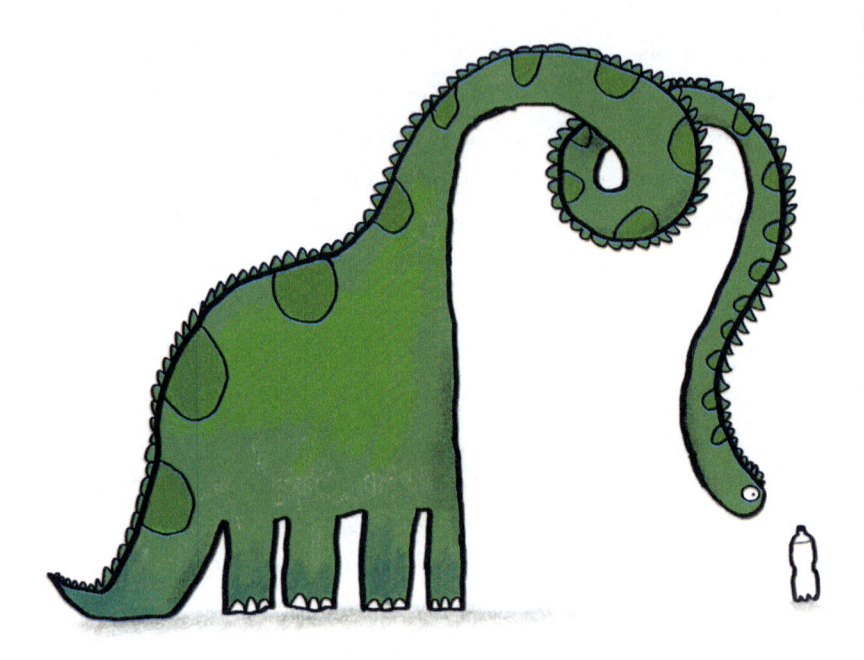

Don't get thirsty

For a nutrient that is so essential to life, water remains remarkably underestimated by most people when it comes to their health. Water is needed to both transport nutrients and oxygen *to* our cells, and to flush metabolic waste *from* our cells, and without it we would simply cease to be.

Water keeps our digestion functioning, our skin healthy, our brains agile and our blood pumping freely, but how much do we actually need? Studies from Aberdeen University show that, on average, 1.5 – 1.8 litres (6-7 glasses) of water per day is more than enough, especially if we are eating plenty of fruit and vegetables.

Pay attention to thirst cues (dry mouth, headache, tension), particularly when older when these sensations become blunted. Add cucumber, mint, citrus or strawberries to water to make it more interesting and always use a good quality water filter as dangerous 'forever' chemicals – ones that don't break down in the environment *or* our bodies – are present in both tap and bottled water. Avoid drinking too much water with meals as it dilutes gastric juices, and ice-cold water can slow down digestion and cause bloating.

> **Did you know?...** There is the same amount of water on planet earth as there was when it was formed. Due to the water cycle, there is an extraordinary chance that the water in your glass is the same water that dinosaurs were drinking 65 million years ago.

32 Noonie Zand Goodarzi

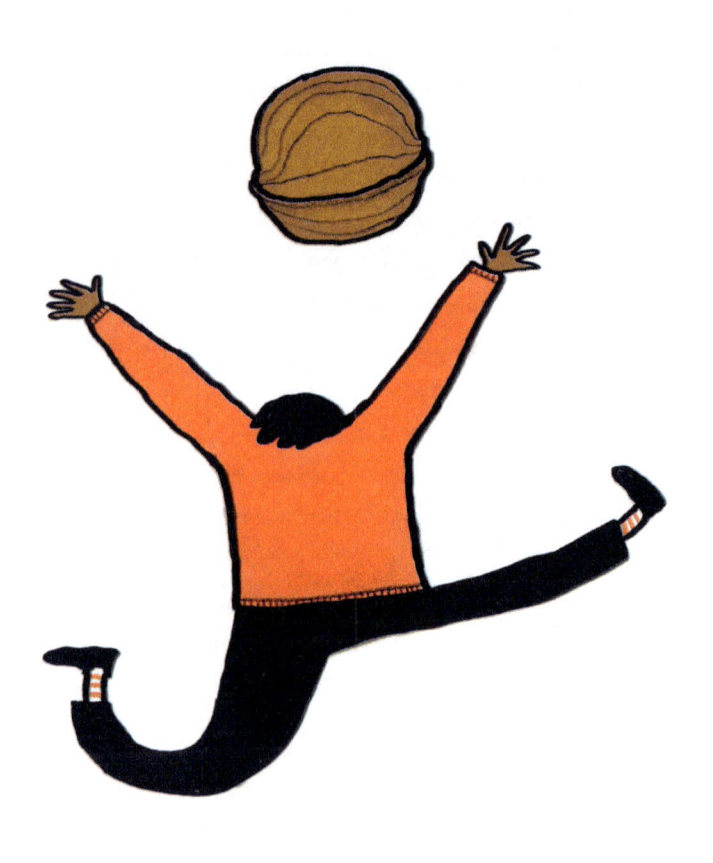

Feel free to go nuts

Nuts are the perfect power food. Study after study has shown that people who eat nuts every day tend to live longer and suffer fewer deaths from cancer, heart disease and respiratory disease.

This is because nuts contain healthy omega-6 fats, plus good amounts of vitamin E, fibre and protein, and their oils help us to absorb nutrients from vegetables. Of all the nuts, walnuts are undoubtedly the healthiest. They have the highest antioxidant and omega-3 levels and one large trial showed that people who ate more than three servings of walnuts per week cut their risk of dying of cancer in half.

Many people hold back on nuts for fear of weight gain, and although nuts are calorific, research has shown that they can increase fat-burning metabolism, causing you to actually lose weight. Have a handful a day of mixed (unsalted, raw) nuts and make sure they haven't been sitting around for too long as rancid oils are harmful. Use in sauces, smoothies and soups; chop up raw into vegetable dishes and salads; pair nut butters with fruit as a pudding or snack.

Did you know?...The Brazil nut tree grows up to 50 metres tall and its nuts can only be gathered once they've fallen to the forest floor. Its flowers are also shaped in such a way that only specific bees can pollinate them.

Noonie Zand Goodarzi

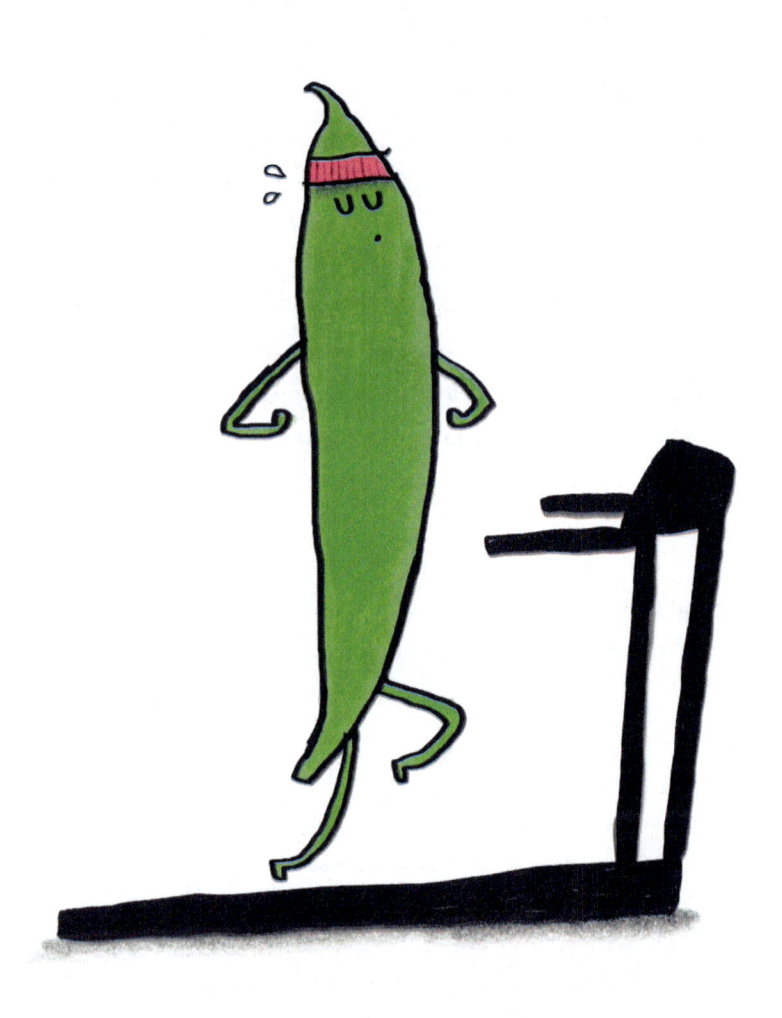

Raise your pulse rate

Pulses are the edible seeds of plants in the legume family and are amongst the oldest cultivated plants. Packed with fibre, anti-inflammatory antioxidants, energy-giving B vitamins, and key minerals magnesium, zinc and calcium, they are the ultimate cheap and easy health food.

Pulses include peas, haricot beans, lentils, chickpeas, cannellini beans, kidney beans, soya beans, black beans, adzuki beans, split peas, butter beans and broad beans… just a few among thousands.

When combined with a wholegrain like brown rice, pulses provide a vegetarian complete protein – containing all the eight amino acids that we need – and, being low in fat and high in fibre, are an excellent means of lowering cholesterol.

Try and have at least one serving a day: a dollop of hummus; a bowl of pea soup; a serving of tofu; a mixed bean salad; some dhal. When sprouted, the antioxidant power of lentils doubles. Sprouts can be added to everything and are not as difficult to make as you might think.

Did you know?... The flatulence-causing compounds in legumes are a type of carbohydrate called oligosaccharides which our gut bacteria break down, producing lots of gas. To prevent post-prandial farting, soak your beans overnight and then discard the water and rinse several times.

36 Noonie Zand Goodarzi

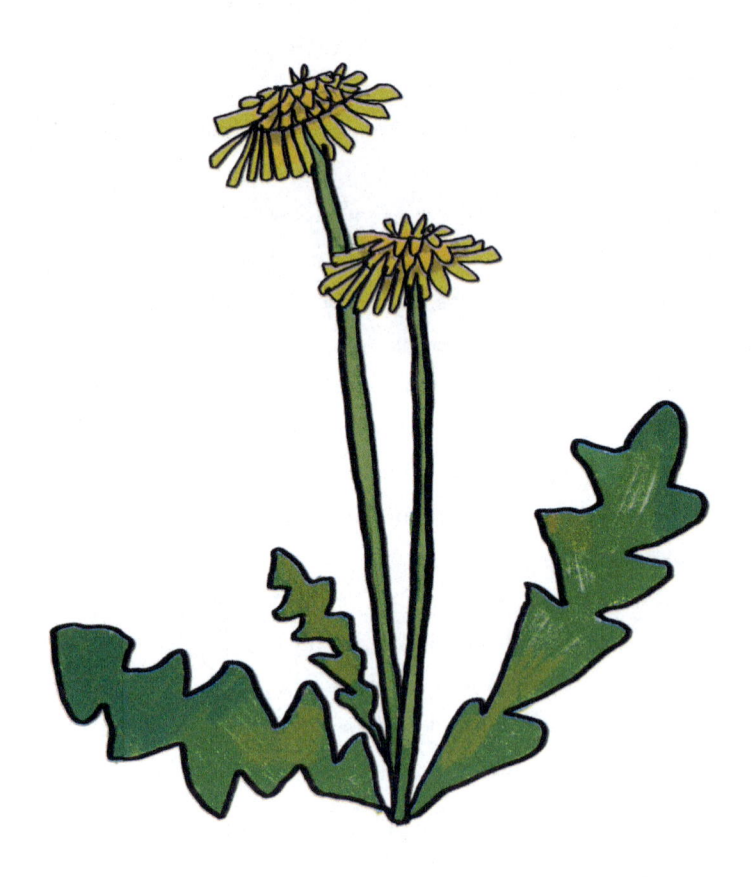

Think bitters for bile flow

Bitter herbs stimulate our bodies to produce bile and, in doing so, give our livers a much-needed boost.

Bile is a digestive secretion released by the liver and stored in the gallbladder. It is essential to the digestion and absorption of fats and important fat-soluble vitamins A, D, E & K; plus it is a safe carrier of toxins out of the body. If bile flow is inhibited for any reason – often due to impaired liver function – toxins will stay in the liver for longer with damaging effects.

Certain foods stimulate bile flow, and it is wise to include them in your diet daily: beetroot, artichokes, radishes, and bitter leafy greens like watercress, parsley, dandelion, chicory, endive and rocket. Spices like turmeric and ginger will also do the job, as do organic acids from apple cider vinegar, lemons and limes.

Start the day with a glass of warm water with the juice of half a lemon (or 1 tablespoon of apple cider vinegar) to stimulate gastric juices including bile flow. Swedish Bitters are good too. They can aid digestion and help relieve gas and bloating.

> **Did you know?**…In the Middle Ages, mystical qualities were attributed to gallstones. Pigmented stones from oxen were used by painters, alchemists and apothecaries, and the gallstones of hedgehogs were prized for their supposed ability to drive poisons out from the body.

Noonie Zand Goodarzi

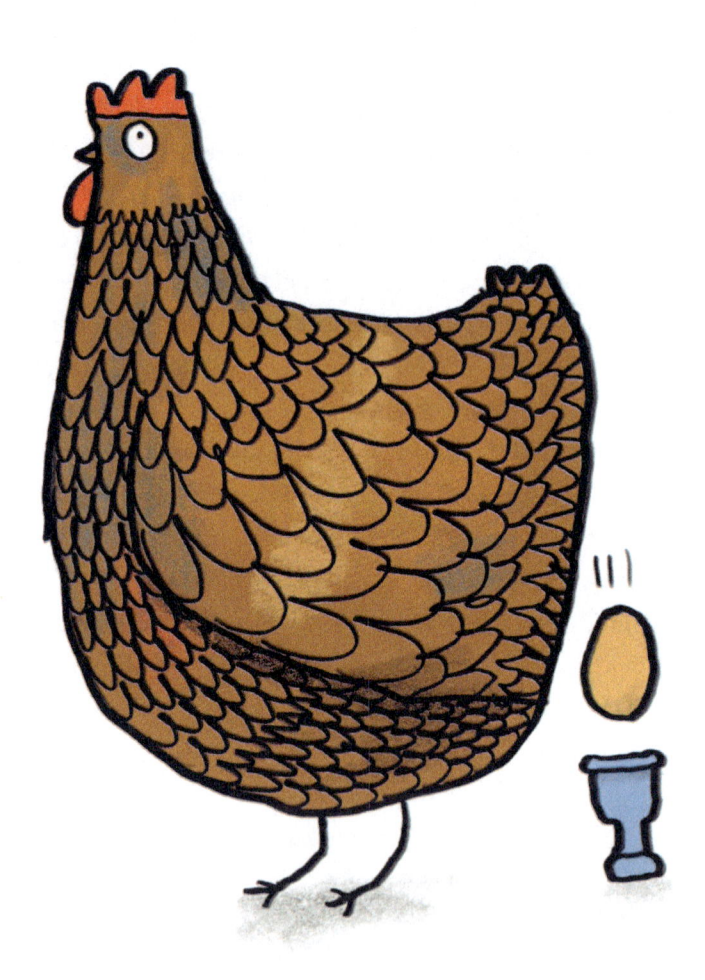

Go to work on an egg

Since the domestication of the chicken, eggs are eaten in almost every country in the world – the reason being that they are an easy, low-cost means of a square meal.

Eggs are the perfect little package, containing protein, antioxidants lutein and zeaxanthin, healthy essential fats, vitamin B12, selenium and fat-soluble vitamins A,D,E,K. In the past, people were concerned that the cholesterol in eggs could contribute to heart disease, but recent science shows that it has no effect on blood cholesterol.

The other controversial component of eggs is choline – an essential nutrient that is important for liver detoxification and brain health. Studies have noticed a correlation between high choline levels and the progression of prostate cancer, so it is recommended to avoid too many eggs in this instance. Otherwise, an egg a day is fine – though I am a firm believer in rotating foods and having days off.

Choose organic free-range eggs from chickens that haven't been fed antibiotics or GMO corn or soy, and look for omega-3 supplemented eggs which contain healthier fats.

Did you know?...Whale sharks are the planet's largest egg-laying animals. These gigantic fish are ovoviviparous which means their babies develop in membranous shells, shedded before birth. The bee hummingbird lays the smallest egg, the size of a grain of rice.

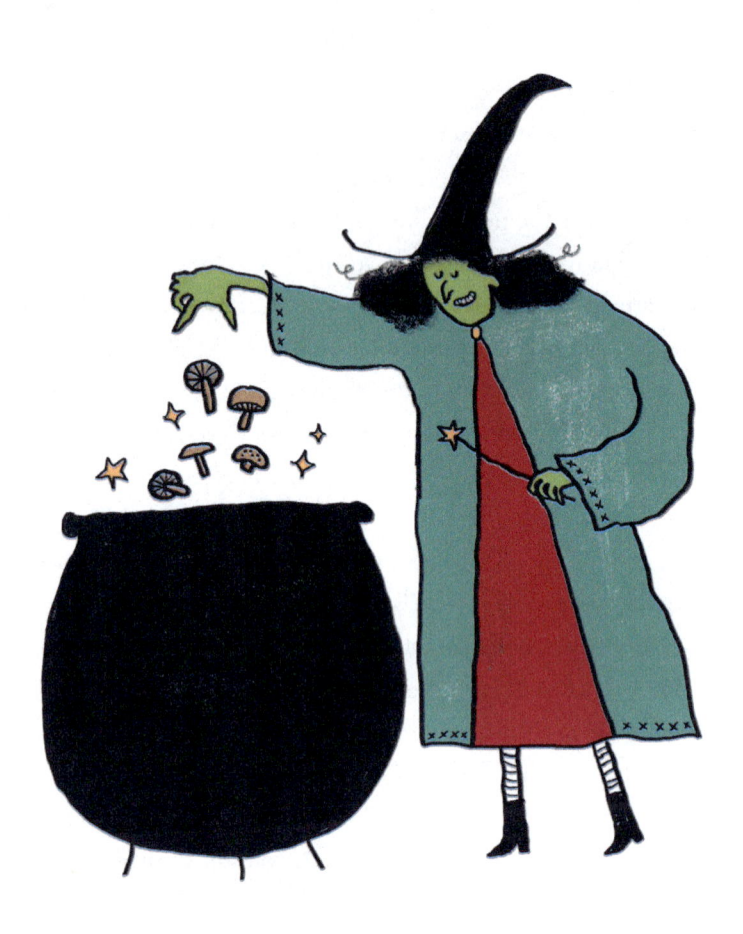

Feel the magic of mushrooming

Mushrooms have long been valued for their beneficial properties in Japan and China, and today functional mushrooms like the mighty chaga, lion's mane, reishi, cordyceps and shiitake feature in alternative coffees and other supplemental powders.

The reason for this is that mushrooms go beyond simple nutrition, standing instead at the threshold of medicine. Active compounds in mushrooms like beta-glucans and ergothioneine have astounding disease-busting benefits. Researchers have found that ergothioneine can protect the DNA in our cells, and because we have evolved a means of absorbing it, it likely plays an essential physiological role.

This compound must be taken in via the diet and the best source by far is mushrooms – particularly oyster, shiitake, maitake, lion's mane, reishi, turkey tail, and cep. Use mushrooms liberally in stir-fries, stews, soups, broths, risotto, gravy, and noodle or pasta dishes. Avoid eating them raw as they contain a toxin that is neutralised when heated.

> **Did you know?...** Mushrooms – or the kingdom of fungi – are more closely related to humans than to bacteria. Scientists believe that humans and fungi shared a common ancestor around 1.3 billion years ago. The mind boggles.

Noonie Zand Goodarzi

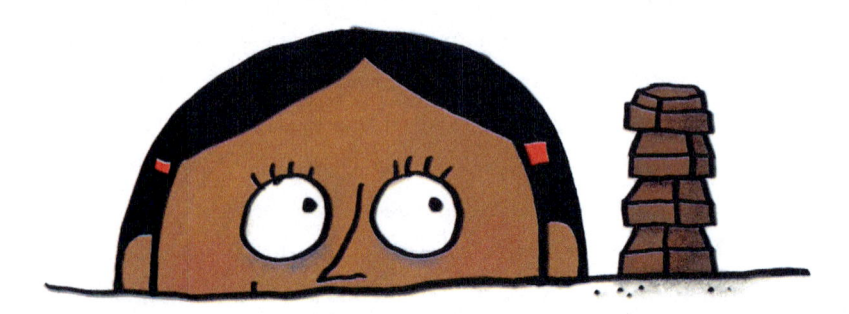

Get your kicks from chocolate

The cocoa content in chocolate is what distinguishes the good stuff from the bad stuff: the higher the cocoa solids, the lower the sugar and milk, and so any bar offering 70% or more cocoa is what you should look for.

Milk chocolate offers pitiful amounts of anything worthwhile and white chocolate doesn't deserve the name, but the benefits of dark chocolate – particularly raw chocolate – are altogether different. Cocoa is surprisingly packed with fibre, plus B vitamins, magnesium, iron and zinc – and its antioxidant levels are higher than blueberries.

Dark chocolate is known to give you a mental boost and that's because cocoa can improve blood flow to the brain. It also promotes the release of endorphins and the production of serotonin, and the theobromine in it increases energy and alertness. Definitely something to be savoured at the end of a meal, but watch out for its caffeine content which can exacerbate heartburn – three small squares of 70% dark chocolate offer roughly the same caffeine as a cup of green tea.

Did you know?... Cacao beans were first used during sacred rituals by the Aztecs and Mayans to make a spicy, bitter elixir to help people attain higher states of consciousness. Aztec emperor Montezuma II allegedly drank gallons of it every day to increase his sexual prowess.

Noonie Zand Goodarzi

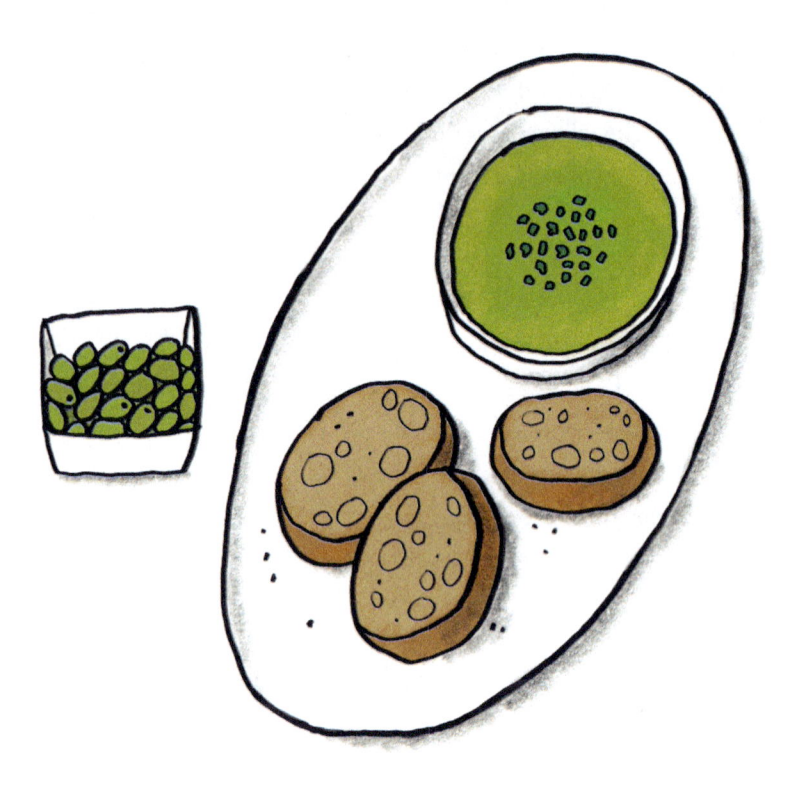

Be generous with the olive oil

If you've ever been to Greece, or any other country that adopts the healthy Mediterranean diet, you'll know how important olive oil is to every meal. Vegetables are cooked with it, salads are drenched in it, bread is dipped in it, and there is always a bottle on the table so you can add even more.

Good olive oil is mostly composed of omega-9 fatty acids which raise levels of good HDL cholesterol and boost metabolism. It is also anti-inflammatory and has a high antioxidant content that can lower the risk of heart disease, cancer and dementia

When buying olive oil, choose cold-pressed and extra virgin, otherwise it will likely have been heated to high temperatures and stripped of nutrients. Look for green and cloudy oils that give a kick to the back of the throat. As it is mainly monounsaturated and full of polyphenol antioxidants, olive oil can be heated without damaging it, though it is best to lower cooking temperatures by adding water, wine or stock; and use it raw liberally.

Did you know?... Greeks consume more olive oil than any another country – an average of 20 litres per person annually. Spain is around 14 litres, and Italy around 11 litres, while the Brits consume about 1 litre per person.

46   Noonie Zand Goodarzi

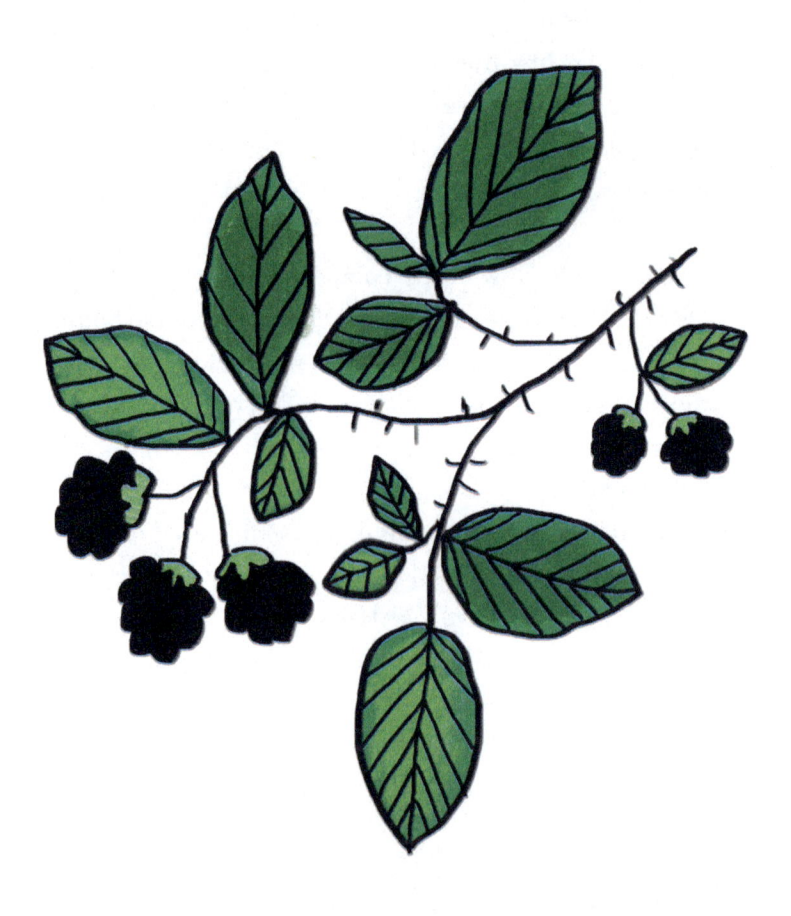

Reap the benefits of berries

Berries are like nature's sweeties – beautiful little jewels filled with anthocyanin pigment, giving them their array of deep purples, blues and reds, plus their superior nutritional powers.

Blackberries, raspberries, blueberries, bilberries, mulberries, strawberries are one of the best ways of obtaining valuable antioxidants. Anthocyanins are nearly twenty times more effective at neutralising damaging chemicals in the body called free radicals than vitamin C and, best of all, they can cross the blood-brain barrier and prevent inflammation in the brain.

If you've ever eaten a mulberry straight from the tree, you'll know how stained your hands and mouth looks after eating it – a true sign of its power. A wild little bilberry or blackberry is much more potent than a shop-bought version so forage as much as you can and freeze your spoils. Also, buy berries in season as it's more likely they were picked when ripe, when antioxidant levels are at their peak. Have a large handful daily.

Did you know?... According to research, people who eat at least two servings of berries a week have a 23% less chance of developing brain disorders such as Parkinson's disease than those who don't.

48 Noonie Zand Goodarzi

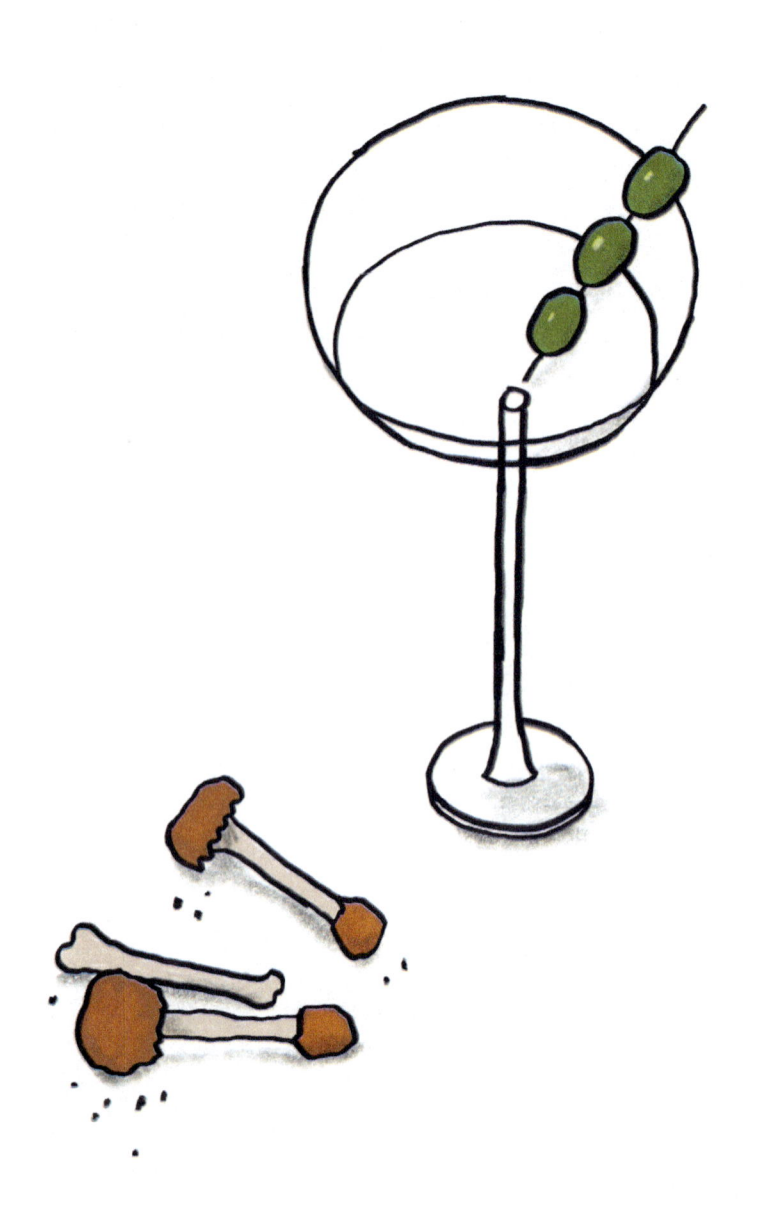

Eat before alcohol

Try as we might, nothing will speed up the rate at which we metabolise alcohol. What we can do, though, is to slow down the rate at which our bodies absorb it, giving our livers valuable time to detoxify.

In general, the less you weigh, the more you will be affected by alcohol, so if you are small, it is doubly important to eat before you drink. Alcohol diffuses through the walls of the stomach quickly so the less food in there, the faster it enters your bloodstream. In fact, peak blood alcohol concentration can be three times higher in people who drink on an empty stomach.

Fried chicken is the perfect pre-drink food as the fat slows the alcohol absorption, plus chicken is high in sulphur-containing amino acids needed in the detoxification process. Alternatives are eggs, salmon, avocado, nuts and seeds. Even if you have just a handful of (unsalted) nuts before you go out, you'd be doing your body a favour. Nuts are also high in B vitamins which are vital to liver detoxification and get used up in the metabolism of alcohol.

Did you know?... Congeners like methanol are chemical by-products of the ageing process of alcohol, and they are the cause of hangovers. Red wine, port and barrel-aged dark spirits like brandy, dark tequila and whisky have more congeners than clear spirits like white rum, vodka and gin.

Noonie Zand Goodarzi

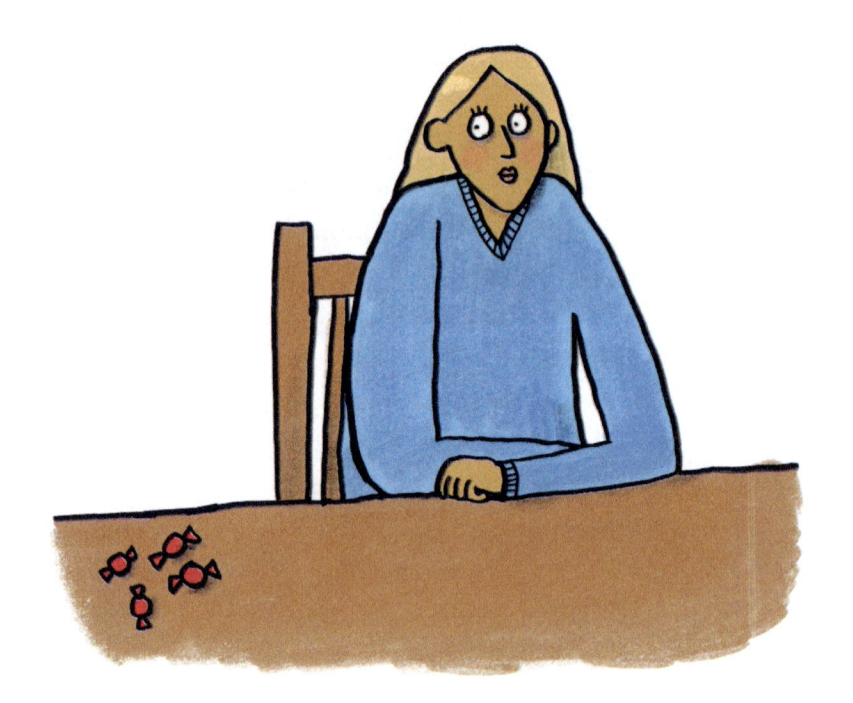

Watch your cravings

When we are tired, stressed or hungover our bodies crave the foods that we think will make us feel better, but afterwards often make us feel worse.

Studies have shown that fat and sugar-filled foods temporarily inhibit activity in the parts of the brain that produce stress and related emotions, and this is why we call them comfort foods. However, be wary of reaching for high-sugar and high-fat foods because the sugar will cause your blood sugar to spike, and the poor-quality fats will simply compound the stress long-term.

We are also usually intolerant of the foods that we crave or have trouble giving up. When we have a mild immune reaction to something we eat, it can act like an endorphin and give us an immediate sense of reward followed by a physiological sense of lack, thus increasing the craving for it. Be mindful of what you find yourself constantly drawn to and see if it correlates with any unexplained symptoms like bloating, mucus or skin rashes.

Did you know?... Cravings can be made worse by stress, boredom and inactivity. Next time you feel a craving for sugar, go for a walk or do some exercise. Drinking a glass of water has also been shown to help – sometimes we mistake hunger for thirst.

Noonie Zand Goodarzi

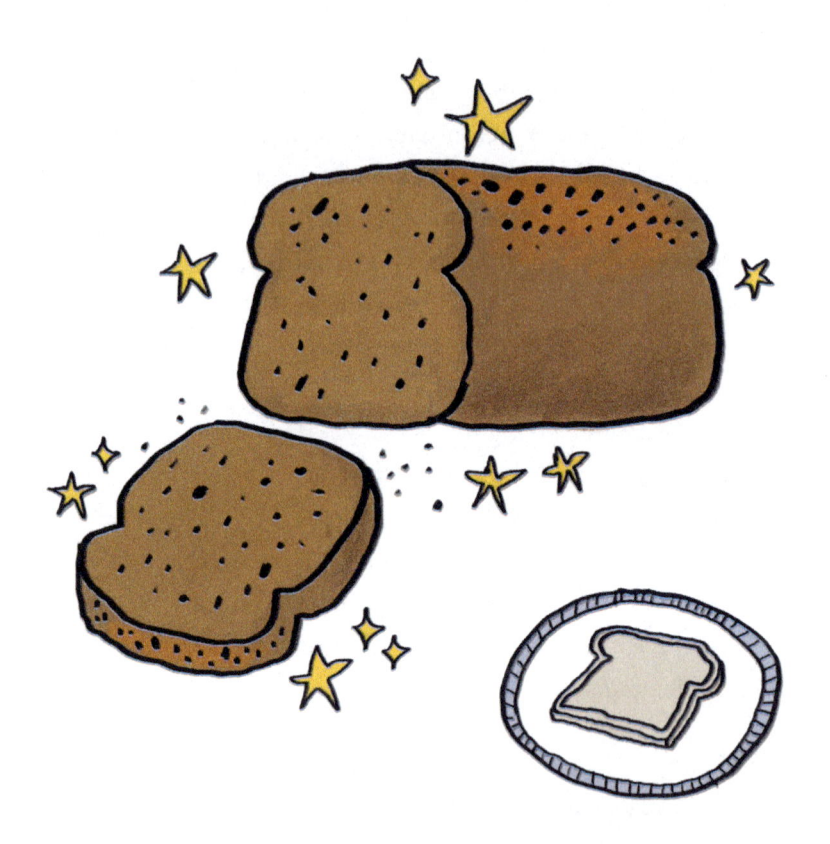

Fill up on fibre

Fibre is one of the secrets to optimum health.

Made up of the carbohydrate part of plants that we cannot digest, fibre ends up in the large intestine where it gives bulk to stools, absorbing toxins and unwanted waste like cholesterol and excess oestrogen and sweeping them out of the body.

Fibre also slows down the release of glucose from food into the bloodstream and provides substrate for good bacteria, thus keeping the gut healthy and happy. For all this, high amounts of fibre have been shown to protect against breast and colon cancer, diabetes, heart disease, obesity… and pretty much death in general!

Humans evolved to eat way more than the 30 grams of fibre per day we are advised to eat today, but even that can be difficult. To increase fibre intake, have vegetables with everything; think wholegrain rather than processed (brown over white); have a handful of nuts/seeds daily; add lentils and beans to stews; eat a salad; choose fruit and dark chocolate for pudding.

Did you know?... 1 slice wholemeal toast contains 2 grams of fibre, 1 cup black beans = 15g, 1 cup lentils = 15g, ½ cup of oats = 8g, 1 apple = 4.5 g, 1 cup raspberries = 8g, 24 almonds = 3.5g, 2 cups kale = 7g, 1 cup green peas = 9g, 1 medium raw carrot = 1.9g, 2 squares of 70% dark chocolate: 3g

54 Noonie Zand Goodarzi

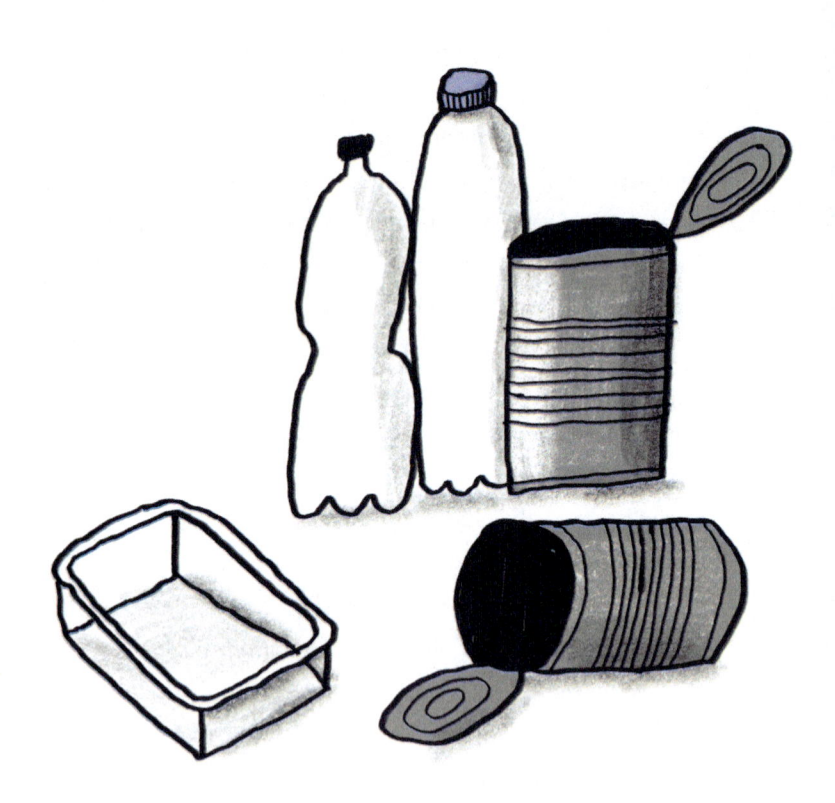

Avoid nasty chemicals

Food is our major source of exposure to toxins – particularly ultra-processed food which has been industrially altered using ingredients that you have not even heard of. Any foods with a long shelf life – like packaged baked goods, fizzy drinks, crisps, sliced bread – are full of chemicals to keep them from spoiling, as well as being packed with sugar, fat or salt to make us want more.

Chemicals are everywhere, so if you can limit your exposure to them, do so. Along with the fertilisers, fungicides, herbicides and pesticides used for growing crops, and the growth factors, hormones and antibiotics used to rear livestock, they are all taking their toll on human health.

New UK government research has found residues of 'forever' chemicals from pesticides (which never break down in the human body) on strawberries, grapes, apples, cherries, spinach, peaches/nectarines and tomatoes – strawberries being particularly bad. Where possible, buy these organic, as washing produce is ineffective at removing residues. Also, avoid cling film, plastic water bottles, storing food in plastic, and filter your tap water.

Did you know?... A common toxin is Bisphenol A (BPA) and Breast Cancer UK is trying to have it banned. It is often found on the inner coating of canned foods and drinks, and its close cousin Bisphenol S is in the shiny coating on till receipts. Choose tetra packs or glass bottles over cans or rinse your canned veg thoroughly; and go receipt-free.

Noonie Zand Goodarzi

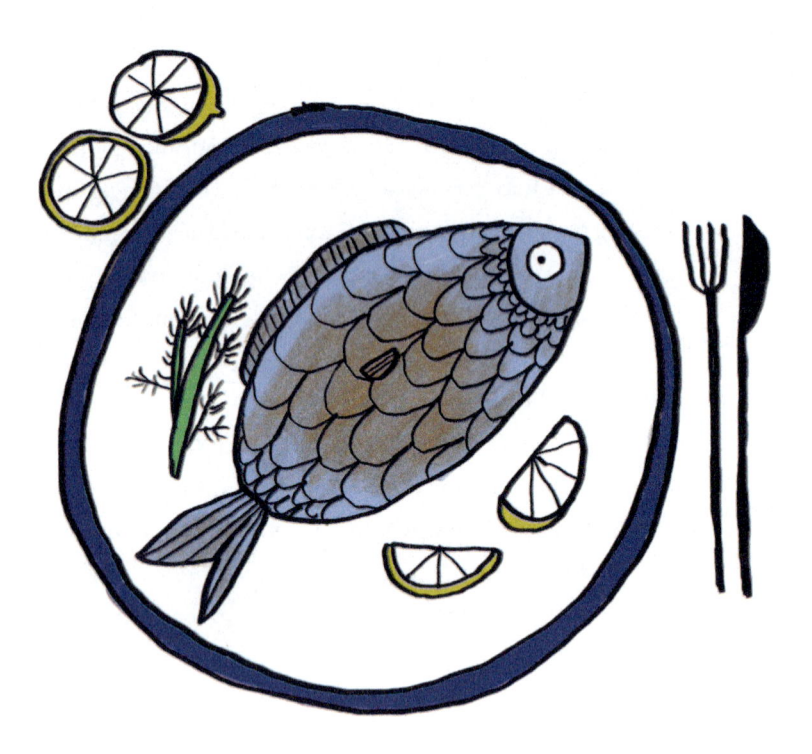

Have a little fishy on a little dishy

Small, wild, oily fish are up there with the best of the superfoods. Mackerel, sardines and anchovies contain lots of anti-inflammatory omega-3 fats which are very important for the health of our brain and our heart.

They also positively affect our cells as, when we eat them, they take the place of unhealthy fats in our cell membranes, keeping them supple and able to let nutrients flow in and toxins flow out. These essential fats are also found in bigger fish such as trout and salmon, though most salmon is farmed and full of antibiotics and should be avoided.

Large fatty fish like tuna and swordfish are also ones to be wary of as their fat contains toxins like mercury. Have some small oily fish 2-3 times a week (tinned versions are a quick and easy option) and, if you buy salmon, save up for the wild-caught Pacific salmon which has the lowest levels of dioxins. Research also suggests that light and skipjack tuna are lower in mercury than larger species like albacore, but it's still not wise to eat tuna regularly.

Did you know?... Pacific salmon return to the same streams used by their parents to reproduce, migrating up to 3,000 kilometres. Scientists believe they can do this due to their unbelievable sense of smell and the particular pheromones found in their home stretch of water.

Noonie Zand Goodarzi

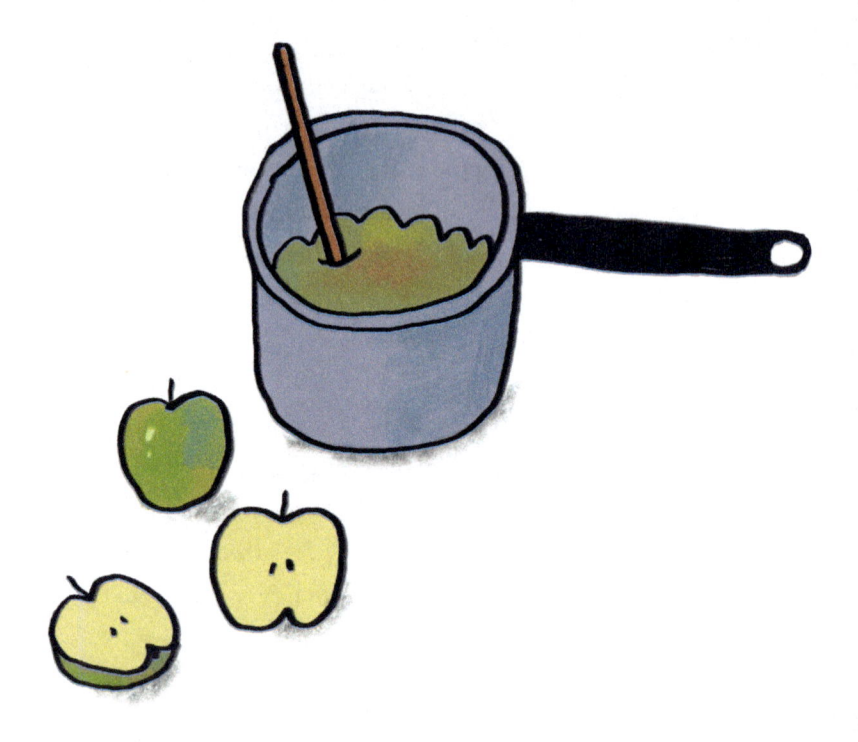

An apple a day

There may be something in the old adage about an apple a day keeping the doctor away, as a study found that daily apple eaters had a 24% lower chance of getting breast cancer, as well as lower risk of ovarian, laryngeal, and colorectal cancers.

Apples are high in antioxidants including quercetin which makes them a good choice for people with allergies, plus they contain soluble fibre called pectin which feeds the microbiome. Stewed apples, in particular, are good for inflammation in the gut as, when cooked, the pectin helps to repair and maintain the lining of the intestine, as well as repopulating healthy gut bacteria.

Don't do as my grandmother did and peel the skin off your apple as that is where all their antioxidants are concentrated, but *do* try to buy organic, as apples are one of the 'Dirty Dozen' – produce with high pesticide residues. Chop into salad or slaws; stew with cinnamon; bake whole; braise with cabbage; or snack on raw.

> **Did you know?...** Apples took off after the Norman conquest when orchards were developed by monks in monastery gardens. Today there are around 7,500 varieties of apples grown worldwide, so it would take over 20 years if you ate one every day.

Noonie Zand Goodarzi

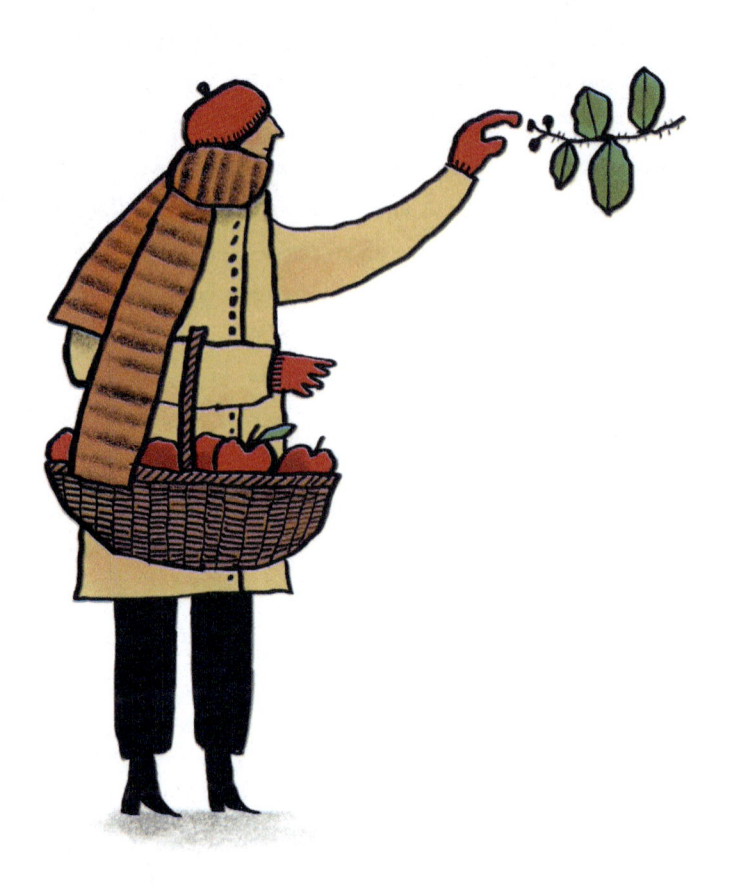

Go wild in the country

Take every chance you can to forage edible plants and berries from the hedgerows. Wild foods are more nutritious than their domesticated cousins because they produce more phytochemicals, or beneficial antioxidants, as part of their defence mechanism against pests and disease – and these are passed onto us when we eat them.

Add dandelion leaves to salads to boost your liver; use nettles in soups or risotto to reduce seasonal allergies; add cleavers to water for lymphatic and kidney health; rose hips are packed full of vitamin C and make a good jelly; wild garlic makes a delicious immune-boosting pesto; add purslane to steamed greens as a boost for your skin; blackberry and apple crumble has huge anti-inflammatory powers, as do wild damsons which are fantastic for jam; elderberries need to be cooked, but their syrup is a powerful immune-booster against winter colds.

Did you know?... Until about 11,000 years ago, with the development of agriculture, humans were foragers. Living in small groups, they shared food and the knowledge of where it grew and, because of this, they are known to have been one of the most egalitarian societies in human history.

Noonie Zand Goodarzi

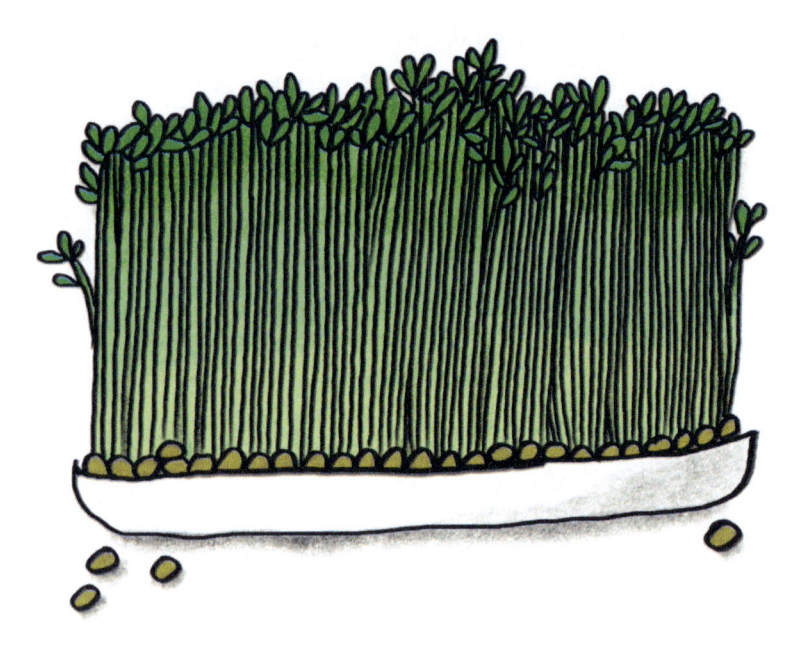

Get sprouting

Sprouted seeds may be little, but they are fierce, and we should include them in our diets at every given opportunity.

When you germinate seeds like broccoli, lentil and alfalfa, they produce small green shoots which can be harvested and eaten. These teeny microgreens contain even more nutrients than their seeds as the germination process unlocks valuable enzymes that make their vitamins, minerals and protein more bioavailable.

Broccoli sprouts contain 100-400 times more of the cancer-busting compound sulforaphane than mature broccoli, whilst lentil sprouts have double the antioxidant power, and chickpeas four times. Alfalfa sprouts are a source of phytoestrogens – plants that can exert both an oestrogenic *and* anti-oestrogenic effect, making them important in the prevention of menopausal symptoms, cancer and heart disease.

Learn how to sprout (basically just a few days of soaking, watering and rinsing) and add them to everything.

> **Did you know?...** Sprouting seeds is an important part of Nowruz, or Persian New Year. At Spring Equinox, people across Iran and Central Asia grow a plate of lentil sprouts or sabzi to symbolically mark the rebirth of nature and the triumph of light over darkness.

64 Noonie Zand Goodarzi

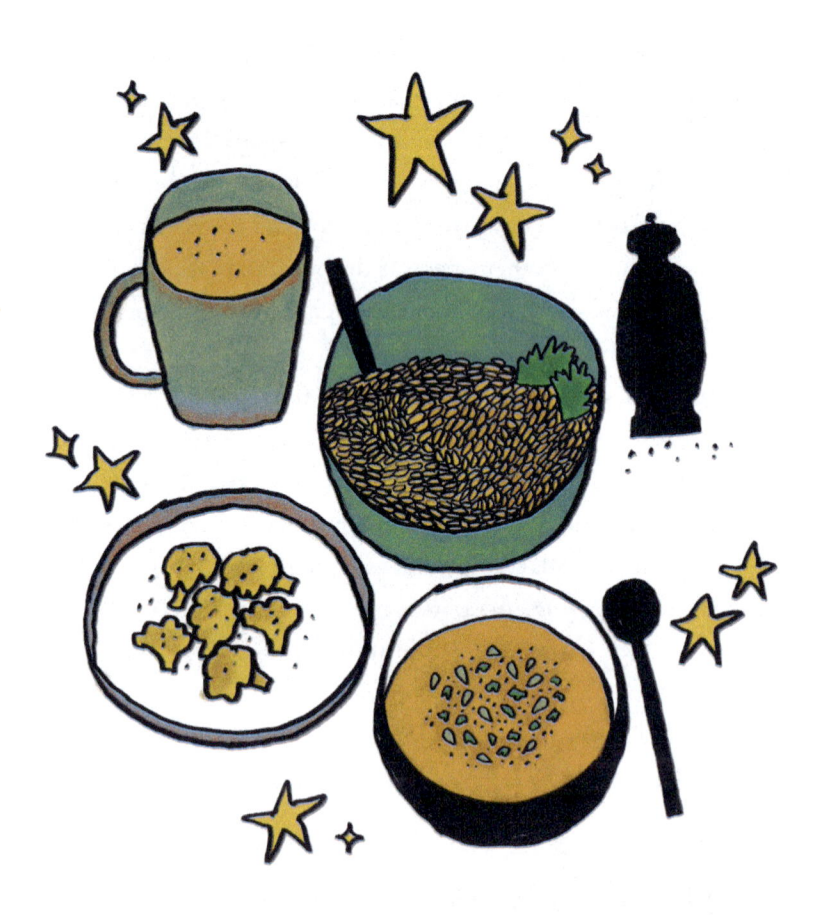

Put out inflammatory fire with turmeric

Inflammation is the seat of all disease and by that, I mean chronic inflammation – a silent, low-grade simmering of immune activity that can go on for years and accelerate ageing. Each individual has their own innate ability to deal with this underlying imbalance, but as we get older the immune system finds the equilibrium harder to hold.

One of the best choices you can make for your health is to adopt an anti-inflammatory diet and to make the spice turmeric central to it. This magic golden root with its bitter, peppery taste and bright yellow pigment, curcumin, has powerful anti-inflammatory properties. Trials have shown its effects comparable to hydrocortisone and ibuprofen, with positive outcomes when used with rheumatoid arthritis and inflammatory bowel disease.

Add it to soups, rice dishes, roasted cauliflower, lentil, bean or meat stews, or make a cup of golden milk – recipes for it abound. Don't forget, combining turmeric with black pepper can increase the bioavailability of curcumin by 2000%, as can, to a lesser degree, combining it with some fat.

> **Did you know?...** Any illness that has 'itis' on the end of its name means there is inflammation involved – 'itis' simply means 'inflammation of'. Arthritis, bronchitis, colitis, dermatitis, encephalitis...and so on through the alphabet.

Noonie Zand Goodarzi

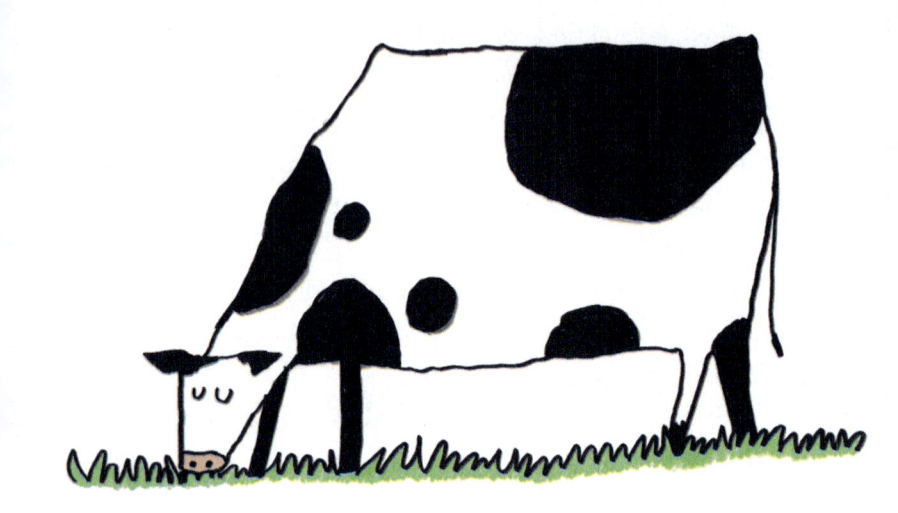

Think twice about processed meats

Sorry to break it to you, but bacon is bad news. Processed meat's link to bowel cancer and cardiovascular disease is well known, but we can now add dementia to the list.

A large longterm study found that by eating meats like bacon just twice a week, you are raising your dementia risk by 14% compared to those who eat it less than three times a month. What is more, each additional daily serving can be linked to increased cognitive ageing. Other than bacon, the worst offenders are sausages, ham, pâté, hot dogs and salami, which mostly contain nitrites, plus high levels of sodium and saturated fat.

If you want meat, choose beef from cows that have been pasture-fed as it is higher in healthier omega-3 fats and, to counteract its pro-inflammatory effects, make sure you are not holding back on fruit and veg. Also, opt for slower, indirect-heat methods of cooking meat like poaching, stewing, and braising, as the higher the temperatures (from frying and particularly barbecuing), the unhealthier the chemical compounds produced in the meat.

Did you know?... Processed meats are categorised as Group 1 Carcinogens. This puts them in the same category as cigarettes and asbestos for their risk of causing cancer.

Noonie Zand Goodarzi

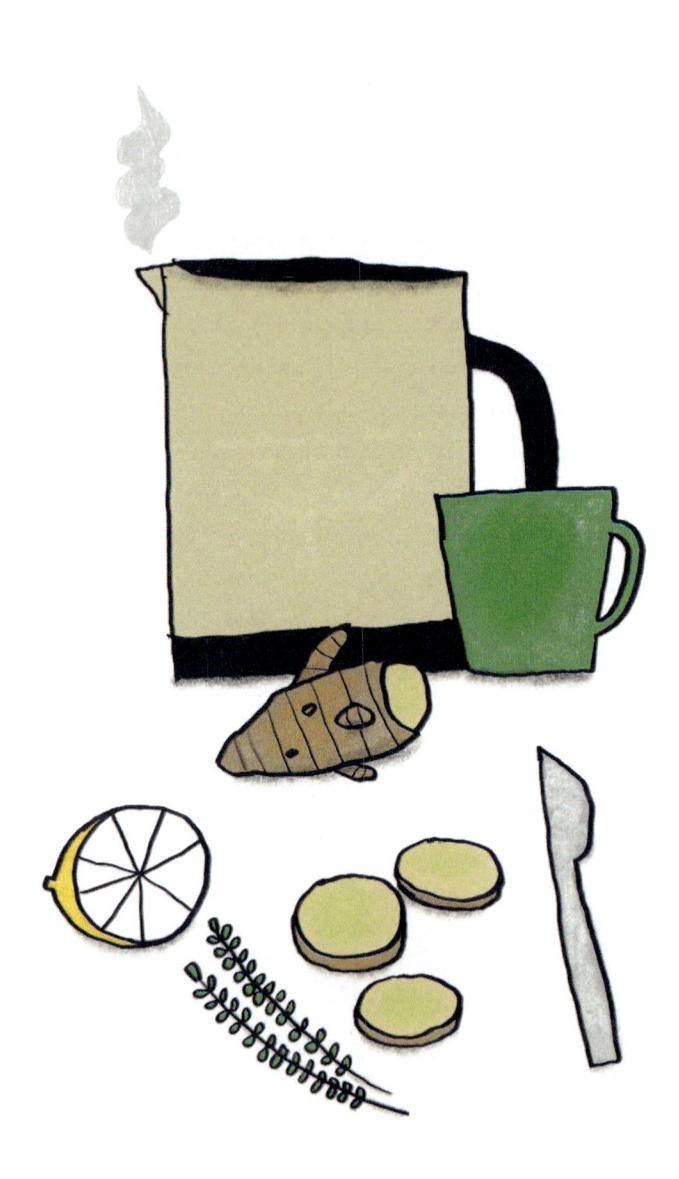

Appreciate the genius of ginger

Ginger should be made a legal requirement. Its fiery taste comes down to the root's gingerol compound which acts as an intestinal spasmolytic, relaxing the gut, encouraging intestinal motility, helping with bloating and wind, plus easing nausea.

Ginger also has powerful anti-inflammatory properties and lesser-known benefits of the root are its treatment of migraines – in a trial just an eighth of a teaspoon of powdered ginger worked as well as a pharmaceutical drug – and its ability to ease painful menstrual cramps.

Ginger tea is a great way to start the day and it is good if you feel a cold coming on. Ginger is diaphoretic which means it will warm you from the inside and promote perspiration. Cut a thumb-sized chunk into small pieces, add three sprigs of fresh thyme, the juice of half a lemon, some honey and hot water – it never fails to help.

> **Did you know?...** Henry VIII, who was terrified of contracting the deadly Sweating Sickness that plagued his realm, recommended eating ginger as a preventive measure against the disease. Not sure if it was down to the ginger, but he never contracted it.

70 Noonie Zand Goodarzi

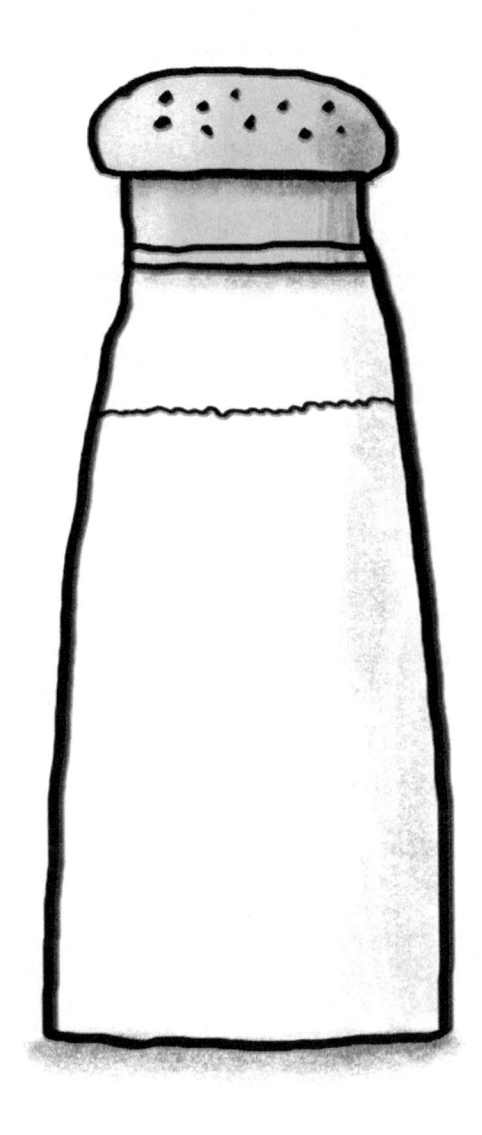

Shake the salt habit

Eating too much salt is one of the major dietary risks for death and disease in the world. We were evolved to get around a quarter of a teaspoon of sodium a day from plants and so our bodies are not built to withstand the high amounts found in the modern diet.

After one salty meal, the sodium-potassium balance in our cells is disrupted, causing water retention, raising blood pressure and, over time, significantly increasing our risk of stroke and heart attack. The British Heart Foundation recommends eating no more than 6g of salt a day (1 level teaspoon), equivalent to 2.5g of sodium, though ideally we should aim lower.

Don't put salt on the table; halve the amount you cook with; avoid high sodium foods like ready meals, sliced bread, processed meat, cheese, pickles, and salty snacks; look for low-sodium soya sauce, miso, ketchup, and stock cubes; flavour with onions, chilli, garlic, lemon juice, and herbs instead. At first, food might taste bland, but after 2-4 weeks your taste buds will adjust.

Did you know?... Salt used to be one of the most important trading goods. In Roman times, salt was so valuable that soldiers were sometimes paid with it instead of money – hence the word 'salary'.

Noonie Zand Goodarzi

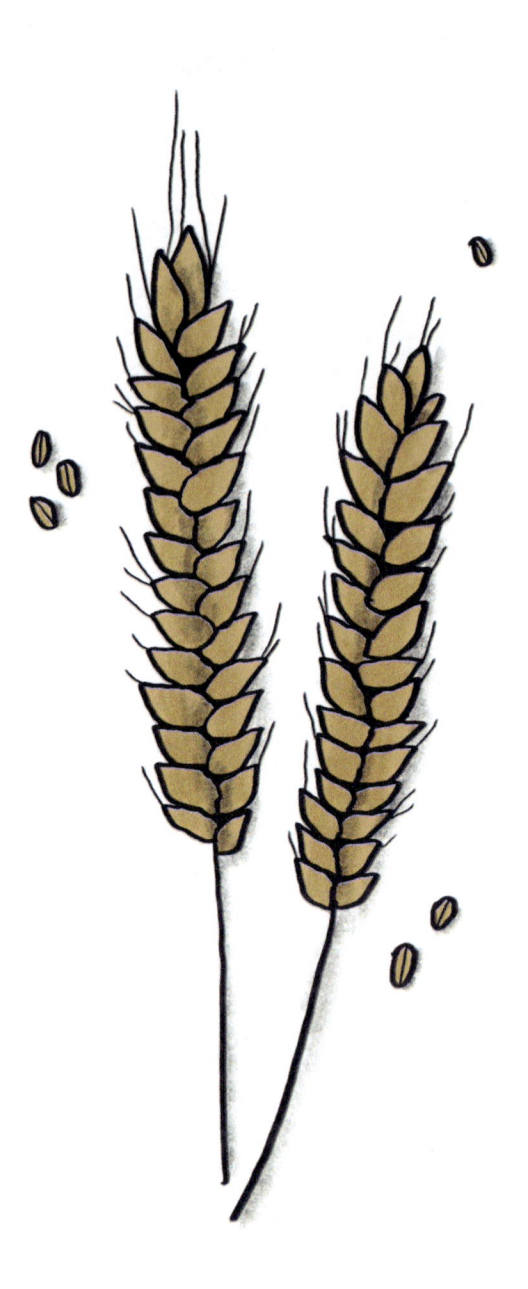

Be wholeheartedly whole grain

Whole grains are exactly what they sound like – the entire grain kernel that hasn't been refined of its bran or germ. Containing more fibre, vitamins and minerals, whole grains in the diet are associated with happier hearts, healthier microbiomes, and an overall lower risk of chronic disease.

Oats are a good example – high in the fibre beta-glucans, they can lower damaging LDL cholesterol; plus they contain an anti-inflammatory compound called avenanthramides that raises levels of the master detoxifier, glutathione. A big bowl of sweetened porridge in the morning can be an assault on your blood sugar despite its high fibre, so make sure that you add protein like nut butter, nuts, or ground flaxseed; and choose steel-cut oats as they are the least processed.

Make the switch from white to brown bread, rice and pasta; and try alternatives to rice and couscous such as quinoa, buckwheat, or millet.

> **Did you know?...** Ancient wheat grains like einkorn and spelt were cultivated in the Middle East up to 10,000 years ago, and were nothing like the over-bred wheat that we eat today. Other early grains were black rice, blue corn, sorghum, teff, millet and amaranth – all gluten-free.

Noonie Zand Goodarzi

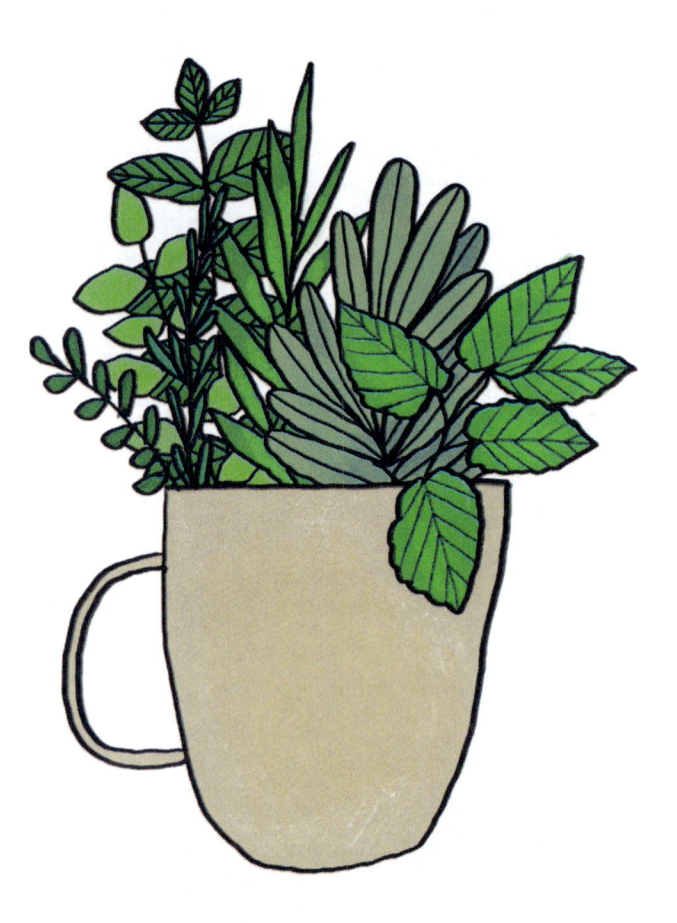

Think herbs and spice and all things nice

Herbs and spices are nature's richest source of disease-busting polyphenols. Just a little pinch in a vegetable dish and a sprinkling in a salad and you are effectively doubling, tripling, quadrupling the health benefits of your food.

The Mediterranean diet commonly makes use of an array of herbs and spices, and it is no coincidence that it is deemed the healthiest diet in the world. Garlic, basil, mint, rosemary, thyme, dill, marjoram, oregano, parsley, fennel, bay leaf, black pepper, coriander, paprika, sage, tarragon, turmeric are just a smattering of what they use to flavour their food.

Surprisingly, it is peppermint which has some of the highest antioxidant levels – great news as you can plant it in the garden and it grows like a weed. Fresh herbs have more goodness than dried ones, but dried are still highly beneficial. Keep your herbs and spices easily accessible and get into the habit of using them *whenever* you can – all the goodness adds up.

> **Did you know?**...The most expensive spice in the world is saffron. Hand-picked from the stigmas of the crocus flower, it takes around 70,000 flowers to get 1lb of saffron and it fetches up to £2,000 per lb.

Noonie Zand Goodarzi

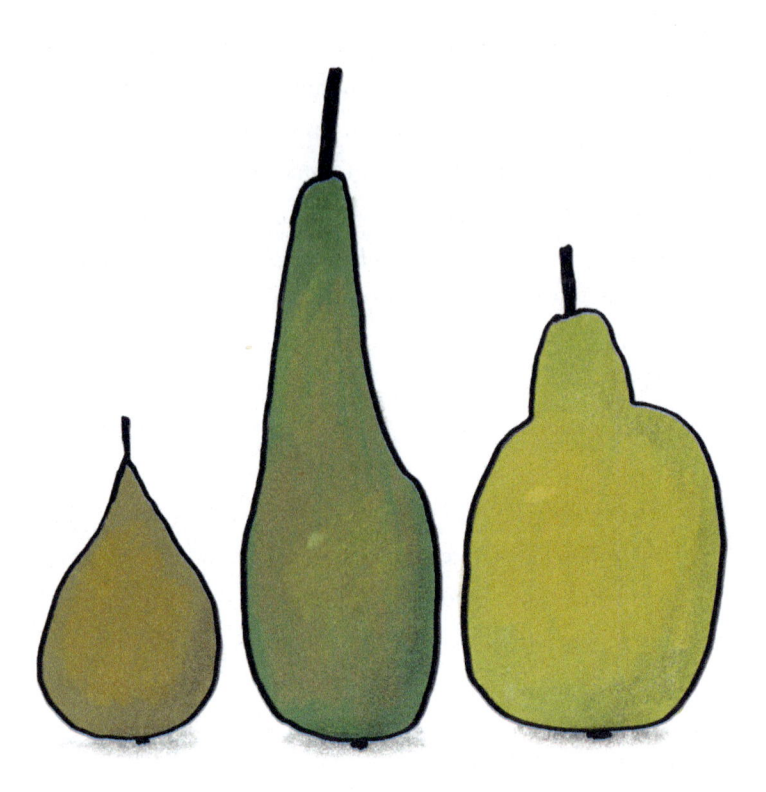

Go pear-shaped

Having a pear body type, with extra fat on the hips and thighs, is considered significantly healthier than if you carry fat around your abdomen.

Larger apple-shaped waists mean that, more than likely, you'll have dangerous visceral fat around your organs which has been shown to raise the risk of diseases like heart disease, cancer and diabetes by as much as 40%. To gauge the risk, measure around the fullest part of the buttocks and then the narrowest part of waist and divide the waist measurement by the hip measurement. A healthy ratio should be 0.8 (ideal is 0.74). Anything greater than 0.85 is associated with health risks and needs to be addressed.

The best thing you can do is to work on reducing sugar and refined carbohydrates and keeping your blood sugar balanced, as excess blood sugar is stored as fat around our middles.

> **Did you know?**...Out of a study of 6,000 women's body types, 46 per cent fell into the straight or rectangle-shaped body; 20 per cent were pear-shaped; 14 per cent were inverted triangles; and only eight per cent of women were hourglasses.

Noonie Zand Goodarzi

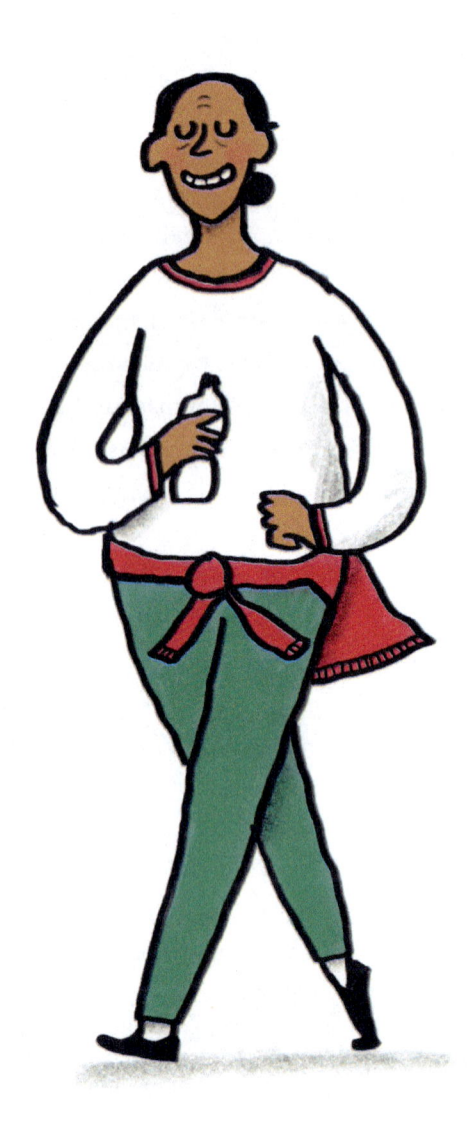

Embrace female-friendly phytoestrogens

Phytoestrogens are natural compounds found in plants that have a chemical structure similar to oestrogen. As a result, they can bind to oestrogen receptors on our cells and, very cleverly, either block the effect of our much stronger oestrogen if levels are too high, *or* exert a mild oestrogenic effect if levels are too low.

These hormone-balancing powers make them useful for women, particularly around menopause when they should be included in the diet daily. They are found in legumes (edamame, lentils, chickpeas); seeds (flaxseed, sesame, sunflower); grains (oats, rice, wheat, barley, rye); fruit (peaches, plums, cherries); veg (broccoli, carrots, rhubarb, celery); sprouts (alfalfa, mung beans); and herbs/spices (garlic, cinnamon, sage, fennel, parsley).

Studies have shown that daily soya intake can halve the severity and frequency of menopausal hot flushes. Avoid highly processed soy protein isolate in favour of whole soy food such as edamame, miso, tofu, tempeh, soybeans and organic soya milk.

> **Did you know?...** Soya in the diet of Asian women has been linked to a 30% lower risk of getting breast cancer compared to US women. Japanese women eat a daily average of 30-50mg of soy whereas American women eat around 3mg.

Noonie Zand Goodarzi

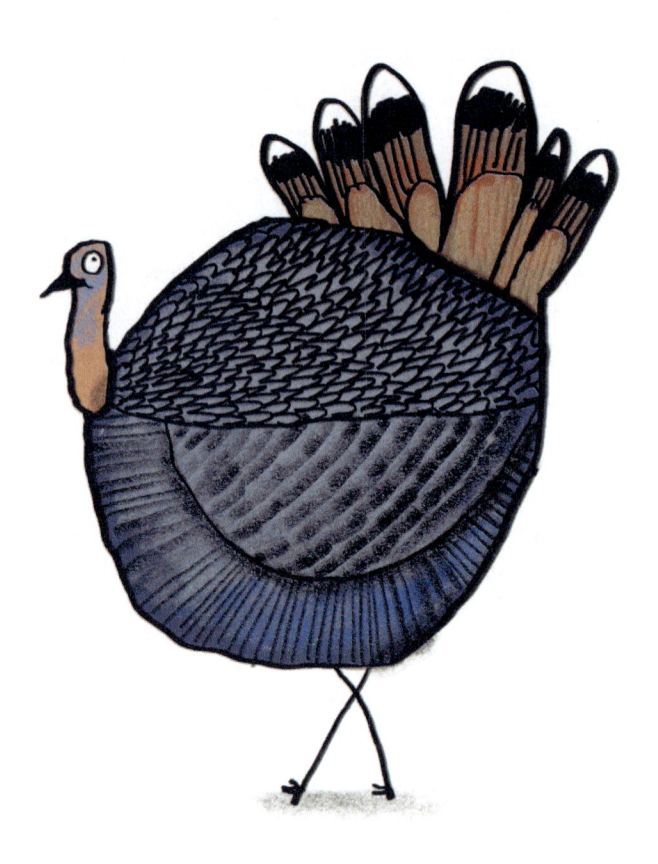

Eat yourself happy

There's a reason why Christmas turkey puts you in a good mood, and it isn't just because of the presents under the tree. Turkey contains the amino acid tryptophan, which gets metabolised in the brain to serotonin – the 'happiness' neurotransmitter that regulates mood, sleep and appetite.

Unfortunately tryptophan's journey through the blood-brain barrier is a notoriously difficult one. It is the least abundant amino acid in any protein we eat, so it has to compete with many other amino acids that have much sharper elbows.

To help tryptophan get to the brain, choose proteins with a higher ratio of tryptophan such as fish, poultry, milk, eggs, tofu, buckwheat, and almonds – and combine them with some carbs which helps clear other amino acids from the bloodstream. Also, make sure that you are getting enough vitamin B6 (turkey, salmon, pistachios, sunflower seeds) and zinc (pumpkin seeds, seafood) which are necessary co-factors for the conversion of tryptophan to serotonin.

Did you know?... Over 95 per cent of the serotonin in our body is produced in the gut. Our gut and brain are in constant communication with the help of the gut microbiome via the vagus nerve, and studies have shown the microbiome capable of influencing mood, cognition, and mental health.

Noonie Zand Goodarzi

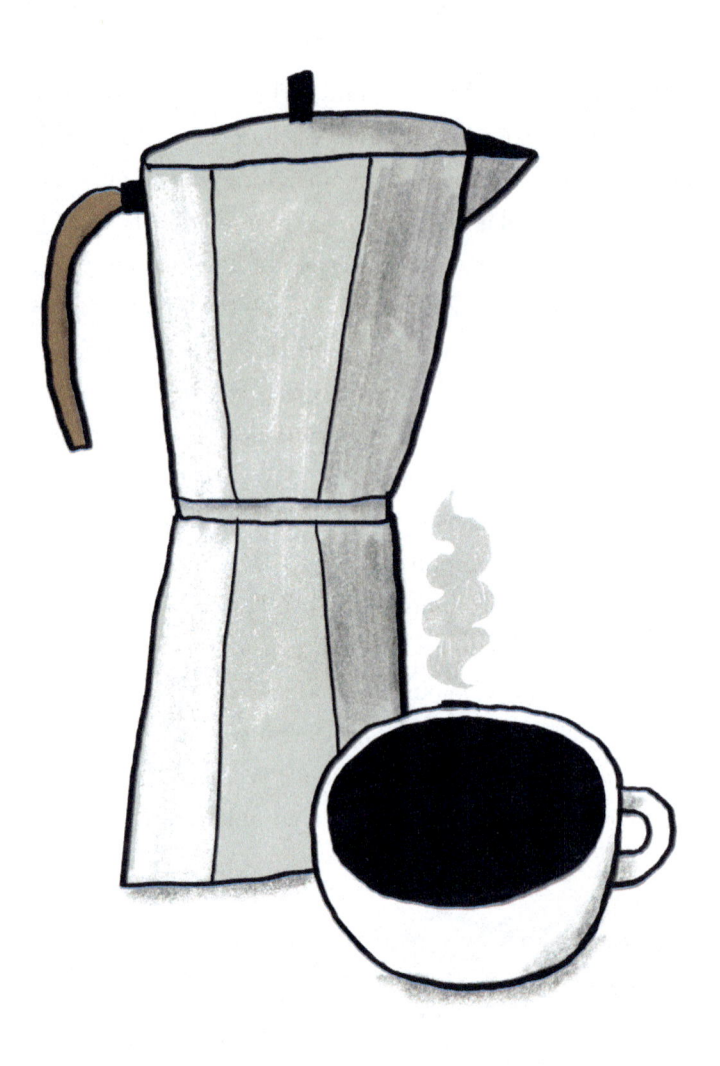

Wake up and smell the coffee

After lots of to-ing and fro-ing, evidence seems to finally suggest that coffee is more healthful than harmful. Considering 98 million cups of the stuff are drunk every day in the UK alone, this is good news.

Coffee contains fibre and prebiotic compounds that feed our microbiomes, plus its anti-inflammatory and antioxidant properties have been shown to benefit diseases of the liver that involve inflammation. Four cups a day appear to be the magic number.

Coffee is not for everyone though. Its caffeine content can exacerbate anxiety, stress and insomnia, plus its acidity makes it not good for people susceptible to gastric issues like reflux. Unfiltered coffee can also raise levels of dangerous LDL cholesterol, so it's best to use a paper filter. Also, if you drink decaf, look for brands that use the Swiss Water method to remove the caffeine, rather than highly toxic chemical solvents like methylene chloride.

Did you know?... Caffeine qualifies as a drug. It is a central nervous system stimulant with a half-life of around six hours. That means, if you have your final coffee at 4pm, half of the caffeine is still in your system at 10pm.

Noonie Zand Goodarzi

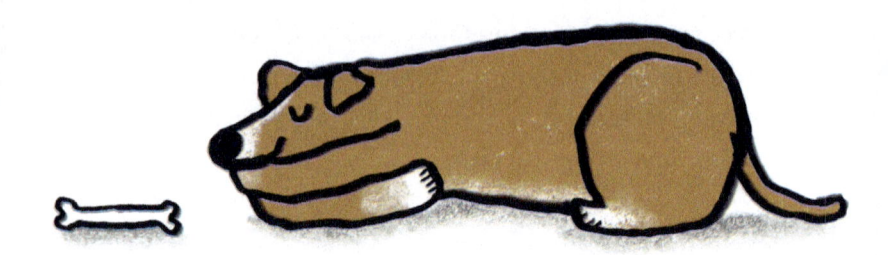

Get well on bone broth

Bone broth – or the clear protein-rich liquid you get from simmering animal bones in water – has been around since man started cooking with fire. Every culture around the world has their version of a broth which is used as a nourishing tonic to promote wellness – particularly if you are coming down with a cold or flu.

The health benefits of broth – which come from amino acids such as glutamine, glycine, and proline – are numerous, particularly in relation to collagen production, intestinal immunity and healing gut inflammation; however, research is still lacking. Nowadays, bone broth has become a popular wellness trend and cartons of it are readily available. Be careful about quality though, as a study found high levels of lead in three types of organic chicken broth.

Bone broth is different from normal stock as cooking time is much longer – around 12 hours. If you have the time and inclination, it is safer to prepare at home where you can be sure of good ingredients.

Did you know?... It appears a 12th-century Jewish physician called Moses Maimonides was responsible for the 'chicken soup as medicine' phenomenon. In his book, *On the Cause of Symptoms*, he claimed that it could cure everything from asthma to leprosy, as well as "rectifying corrupted humors".

Noonie Zand Goodarzi

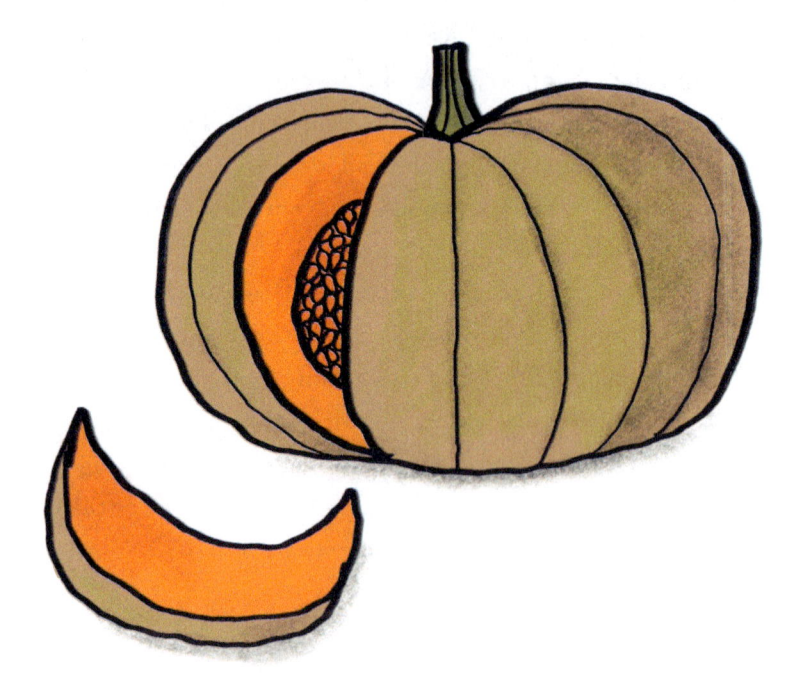

Use pumpkin seeds for prostate health

Pumpkin seeds deserve a special mention as a beneficial plant food for prostate health. These nutty green seeds contain a compound called beta-sisterol which helps to block the conversion of testosterone into a metabolite known to promote prostate growth.

Pumpkin seeds also contain high levels of omega-3 fats, protein, magnesium, beta-carotene, iron, and especially zinc. Zinc is critical to prostate health – the prostate makes more use of zinc than anywhere else in the body, and low levels are common in prostate cancer. Zinc is also central to immune health in general, as all of our white blood cells need it to function, plus it is needed for the detoxification of alcohol – all important reasons to eat these little seeds.

Have them raw or roasted and sprinkle on salads; sauté with carrots or greens; crush and add to biscuits or crumbles; add to mince or veggie burgers; and use as a garnish on soups.

Did you know?... Trying to grow the biggest pumpkin in the world is a serious contest. The current record is held by a Mr Travis Gienger from Minnesota, USA for a pumpkin that weighed 1.25 tonnes – the size of a family car.

88 Noonie Zand Goodarzi

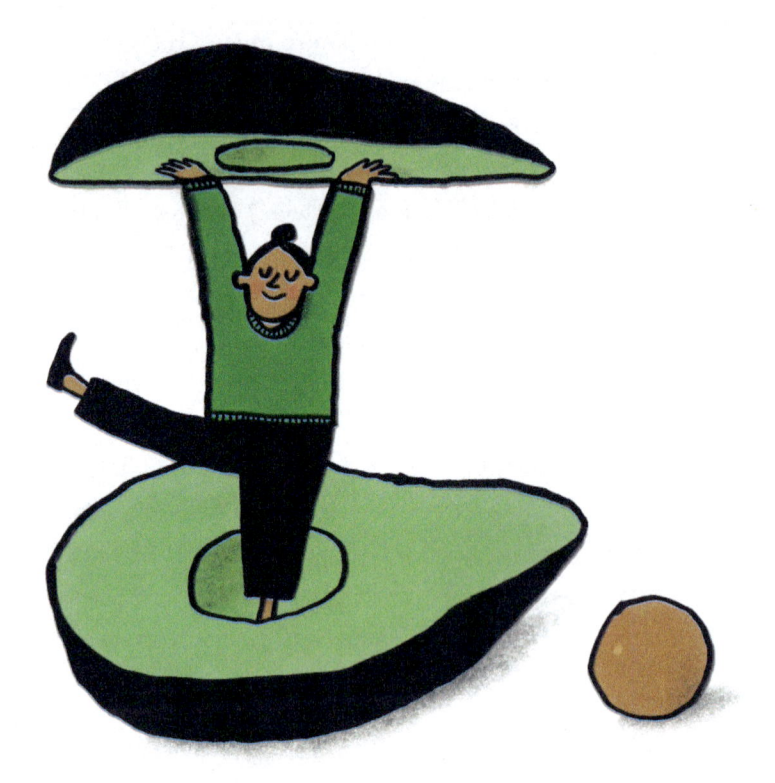

Go guacamole

The avocado has been domesticated for over 10,000 years in Latin America, revered as it was by early indigenous people for its sustenance and power. It is easy to see why this ancient fruit was given near mythical status. An avocado contains lots of antioxidant vitamin E, plus folic acid, potassium, fibre, protein and healthy fats.

Many people worry the buttery consistency of avocados will make them gain weight, but they needn't fear. Over 70% of the fats in avocados are monounsaturated omega-9 fats, similar to olive oil. These fats will actually boost metabolism, and research has shown that instead of putting on weight, women who regularly consume avocados typically have reduced abdominal fat (including dangerous visceral fat around their organs).

If you are an avocado fan, you will also likely be benefitting your cholesterol levels as avocados can raise good HDL and lower bad LDL cholesterol. It's a win-win.

Did you know?... Avocados have a unique ripening process in that they do not ripen until picked from the tree. These fruits can stay on the tree for many months and remain unripe, only beginning to soften when removed from the branch.

Noonie Zand Goodarzi

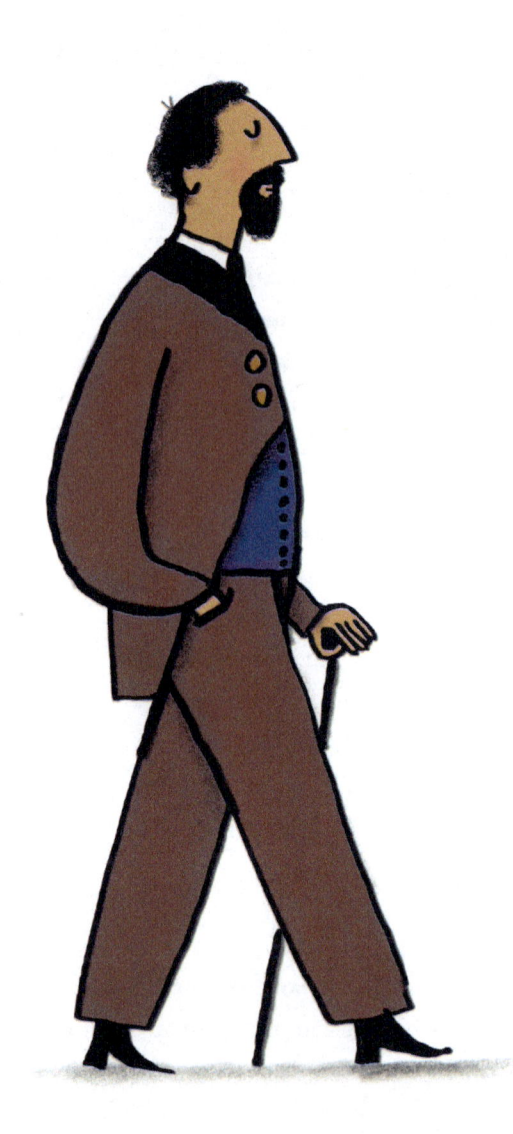

Take a stroll after eating

There is something very worthwhile in the old-fashioned custom of taking a postprandial stroll. Being sedentary for long periods has been called the new smoking, such are the bad effects on your health, and sitting around after a meal is particularly bad.

When we walk, the glucose that is swishing around our bloodstream from the food we've just eaten is shunted into our muscles, where it is used for energy, thus greatly improving our blood sugar levels. Studies have shown that walking – even if it's for just for a few minutes – will have beneficial effects on your blood glucose.

Walking at a late-for-a-train pace for 30 minutes straight after a meal, moreover, has proved very effective for weight loss – more so than sitting around for an hour before you walk. Walking boosts metabolism and benefits digestion, stimulating food to move through the gut more rapidly, thus preventing bloating. All good reasons to get up and move.

Did you know?... Walking wasn't a thing until the late 1700s. Before then, it was seen simply as a necessity and not done unless you were poor, and possibly criminal. The writer Charles Dickens made walking fashionable, known as he was to walk briskly around 12 miles a day.

Noonie Zand Goodarzi

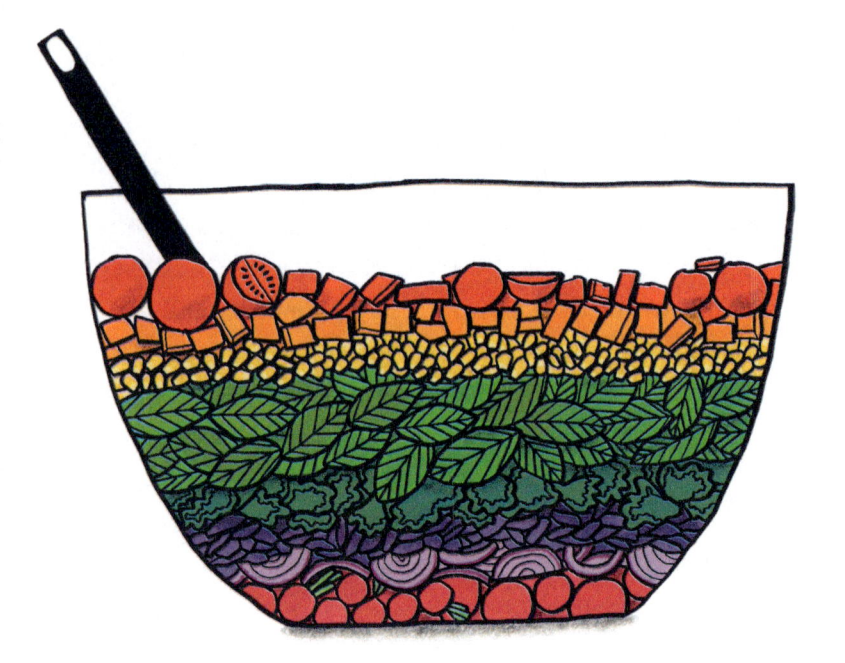

Get creative with salads

Having a salad every day is an easy way of making sure that you are getting a wide range of phytochemicals from fruit and vegetables.

Numerous studies have shown that different vegetables target different cancer cells, so the most effective all-round way of preventing cancer is to have as diversified a diet as possible. Salads are alkaline-forming foods, which our bodies like, and are a source of raw food, which means that no vitamin C or plant enzymes have been lost in the cooking process.

When making a salad, take the salad bar approach and make it as colourful as possible: greens first – spinach, lettuce, bitter leaves like watercress or rocket, herbs like parsley or coriander; then toppings such as beans, berries, nuts, seeds, onion, avocado, tomato, pepper; then the sprouted seeds and fermented veg; and finish it off with a salad dressing made with good olive oil, fresh garlic, and apple cider vinegar… and bam! You've covered just about every nutritional base.

Did you know?... The oldest English language cookbook, *The Forme of Cury* (1390), contains the first known recipe for salad – and look how varied it is: "Take parsley, sage, green garlic, scallions, lettuce, leek, spinach, borage, mints, primroses, violets, porrettes (young leeks), fennel, garden cress, rue, rosemary, purslane; rinse and wash them clean. Peel them. Tear them into small pieces with your hands and mix them well with raw oil; lay on vinegar and salt, and serve."

Noonie Zand Goodarzi

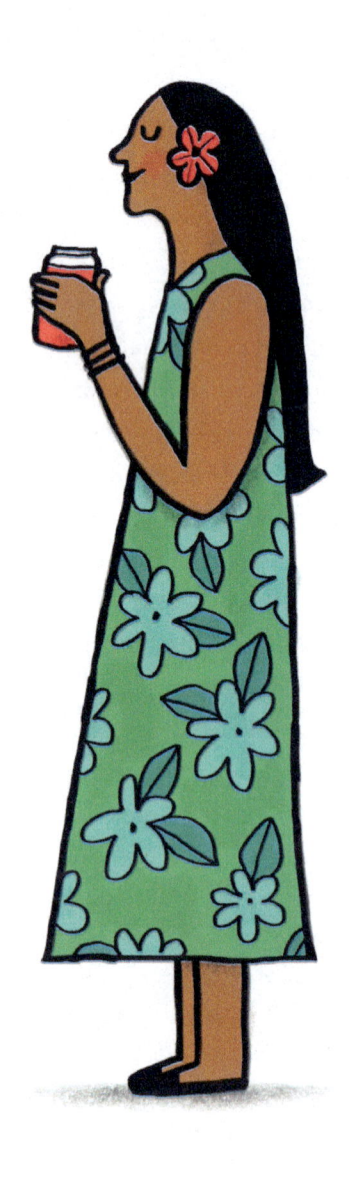

Lower your blood pressure with hibiscus tea

In a trial testing the antioxidant power of 280 common drinks, hibiscus tea came out on top, putting even green tea in the shade.

Hibiscus tea is an infusion made from the beautiful crimson-coloured calyces of the tropical Hibiscus flower. With its lip-smacking tartness and deep red colour, its impressive health benefits should encourage everyone to make it part of their herbal tea collection.

Within an hour of drinking it, antioxidants are absorbed into the bloodstream and then set to work suppressing inflammation – notably in the liver. Another promising effect is hibiscus's ability to lower blood pressure by increasing nitric oxide production which dilates blood vessels. One study showed that two cups of tea daily (made with 5 tea bags) lowered blood pressure by the same amount as the starting dose of a medical drug.

Brew up a batch – Red Zinger is good – and put it in the fridge to drink throughout the day. Do like the Jamaicans do and add ginger to it, and you can sweeten, if needs, with a little raw honey.

> **Did you know?...** In Hawaii, the beautiful trumpet-like Hibiscus flower is often worn behind the ear to show relationship status: the right side for those looking for love and the left for those already spoken for.

Noonie Zand Goodarzi

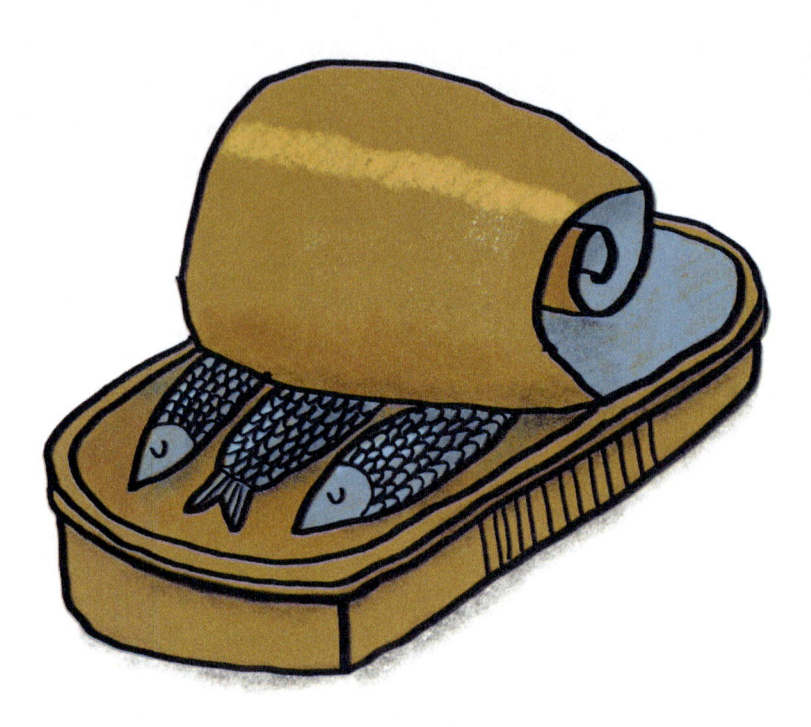

Sort out your fats

Unjustified research in the 1970s made fat into the weight-watcher's nemesis and since then all fats are often tarnished by the same brush.

The thing is, the body absolutely needs some fat from food: for energy production; to absorb fat-soluble nutrients; to build cell membranes and nerve casings; and for blood clotting and muscle movement. However, not all fats are created equal and it's important to know the difference.

In short: saturated animal fats (meat and dairy) are pro-inflammatory and can raise bad cholesterol so should be eaten in moderation; omega-6 fats from nuts and seeds and their oils can be anti – *or* pro-inflammatory depending on your general diet – beware the high sugar/carb diet which shunts them down a pro-inflammatory pathway; eat more anti-inflammatory omega-3 fats from cold water oily fish, flaxseed or walnuts, and include healthy monounsaturated fats like olive oil.

Above all, beware of 'fat free' foods which are usually loaded with compensatory sugar, and avoid trans fats, hydrogenated fats or partially hydrogenated oils which are unsafe in any amount.

> **Did you know?...** When heated, polyunsaturated fats like sunflower oil turn from healthy to harmful, producing toxic aldehydes. Saturated fats like butter are stable, produce no aldehydes when heated, but should be used sparingly. A healthier oil to cook with is olive oil as it contains mostly monounsaturated fats.

Noonie Zand Goodarzi

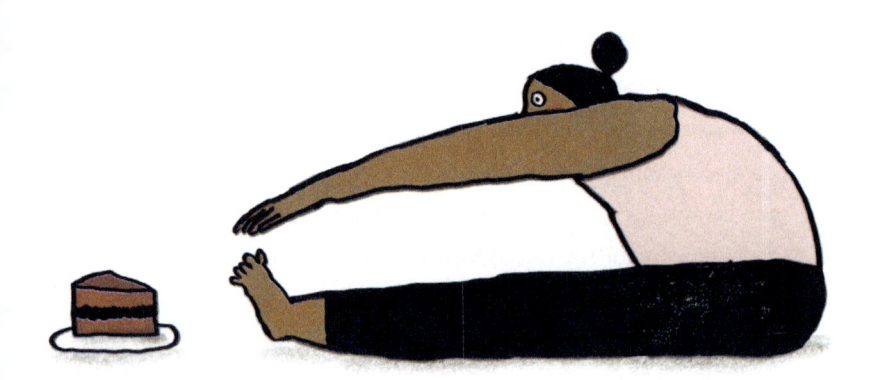

Indulge in a little of what you fancy

The older I get, the more I understand how important it is to remain flexible. Flexible in body, yes, but also flexible in mind, and both of these states are the secret to staying young.

Eating a healthy diet also includes flexibility, and this is sometimes referred to as the 80:20 approach – that is, eating optimally 80% of the time, but allowing yourself a flexible 20 per cent where you can enjoy foods without feeling deprived or forced to fall off the wagon and binge. The occasional treat is a wonderful thing, and we should all allow ourselves them – a bowl of ice cream, a biscuit, a burger – especially if you have made them yourself so you can recognise their ingredients.

Don't get too hung up on the numbers thing either. The general idea is not simply to eat junk 20 per cent of the time – more that you should eat a clean diet for the majority of the time, but if the occasion arises when you are offered a large slice of chocolate cake, then take it….and enjoy it. Restriction can become very unhealthy in itself.

Did you know?... Elizabethans constructed buildings called banqueting houses purely to have their pudding in. One banquet in 1590 refers to a dessert raised to such a "monstrous ticklish height" that it nearly touched the ceiling.

100 Noonie Zand Goodarzi

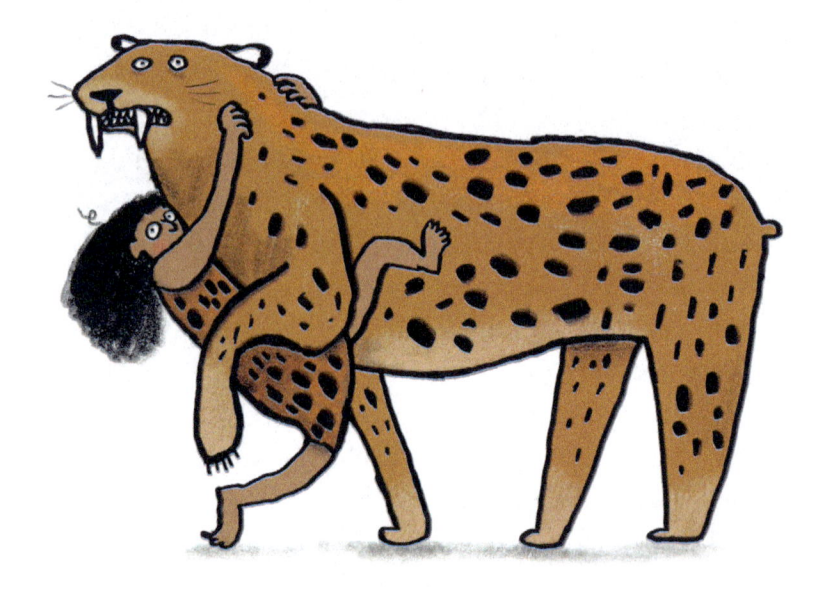

Use adaptogens for stress management

Modern-day stress is out of control and we are simply not built for it. Our ancestors would have had occasional moments of stress (perhaps a wrangle with a sabre-toothed tiger?), but afterwards their body would have quickly recalibrated.

Today, we are so overwhelmed by the pace of life that our stress response is permanently activated, which means higher amounts of the stress hormone cortisol in the bloodstream for longer. If you feel wired but tired, awake unrefreshed, have difficulty sleeping, can't think straight and are running on stimulants, it's likely your cortisol is dysregulated and your adrenals suffering.

Help comes in the form of proper rest, clean diet, therapies such as breathwork, and adaptogens – natural compounds that help us to manage stress, combat fatigue and boost endurance. Good examples are Maca and Ashwagandha. Look at powders or functional coffees (coffee with added superfoods) containing these adaptogenic roots and include them in your diet during periods of high stress.

Did you know?... Mental Health UK's *Burnout Report, 2024* claims that 9 in 10 UK adults experienced high stress in the past year. Almost 25 per cent feel unable to manage stress and 20 per cent needed time off work due to stress, most of them aged 18-24.

Noonie Zand Goodarzi

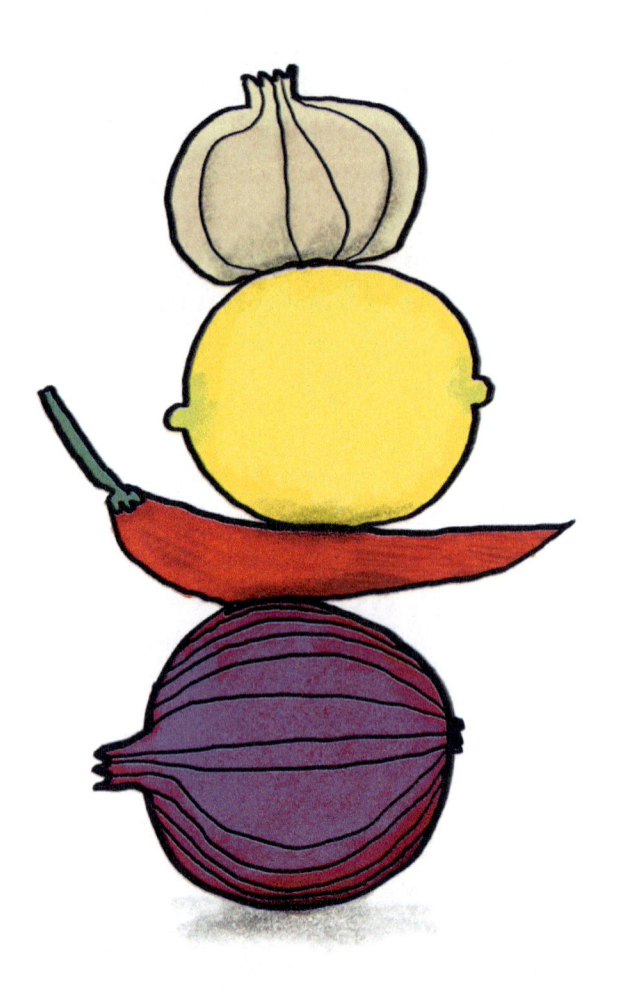

Add in some raw food

A strict raw food diet consists of fruit, vegetables, nuts, seeds, herbs, sea kelp, and cold-pressed oils – essentially whole plant foods that have not been heated above 118 °F (40 °C) and are often sprouted and fermented to preserve enzymes and increase nutrients.

Raw food has enormous benefits to the body: it's anti-ageing; good for the heart and brain; enhances immunity; aids digestion; creates a sharper mind; and boosts energy. It also makes you look fantastic – with clearer skin, brighter eyes and shinier hair – which is probably why it is big in celebrity circles. Raw foodies aim to have 75 per cent of their diet raw, but really any amount is a benefit.

Aim for berries with chia seeds for breakfast, a big salad with sprouted seeds for lunch, a handful of nuts and some raw chocolate for a snack, sauerkraut with your dinner and you're already halfway there.

> **Did you know?...** The Raw Food movement started in the 1800s with a Swiss doctor called Maximilian Oskar Bircher-Benner who believed raw foods contain direct energy from the sun. Bircher-Benner was big on oats, fruit and nuts and gave his name to the famous Bircher muesli.

Noonie Zand Goodarzi

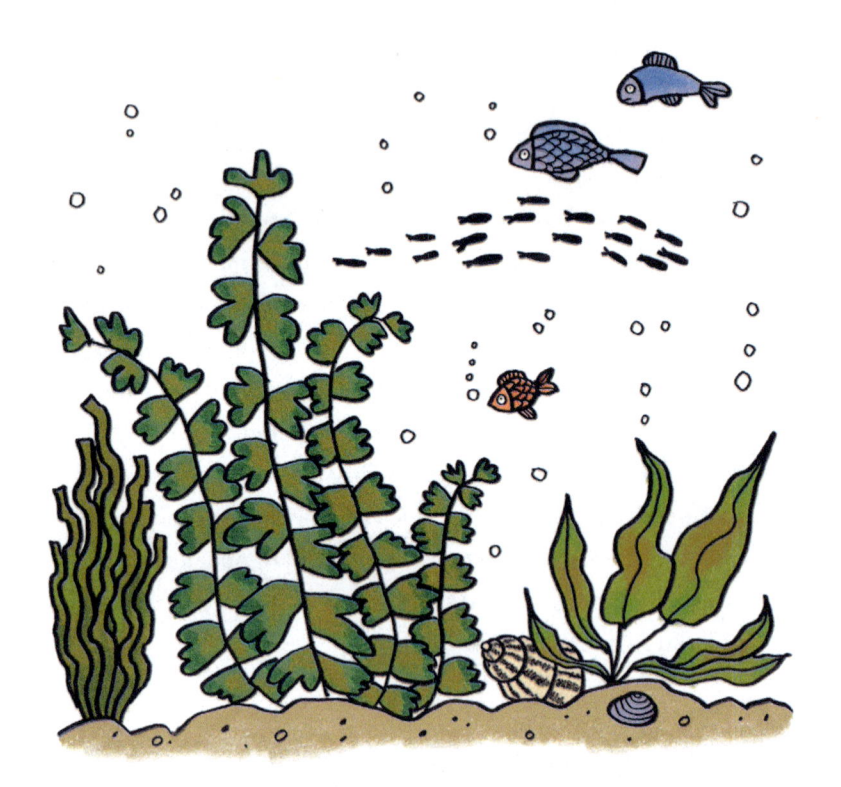

Feed your thyroid

The thyroid is a butterfly-shaped gland that sits in the base of the neck and its importance cannot be over-stated.

Often called the master regulator, the thyroid makes and secretes thyroid hormones that are essential to many bodily processes, including our heartbeat, body temperature, breathing rate, hormone regulation and our metabolism (the process by which we convert food into energy). With such far-ranging effects, it is crucial that we keep our thyroid happy, as an under-functioning thyroid can wreak havoc on our health, commonly causing fatigue, weight gain, brain fog and sluggish digestion.

The thyroid is susceptible to the impact of stress and is needy of certain nutrients, notably: iodine (largely in seafood, edible seaweed, blue-green algae like chlorella and spirulina); selenium (Brazil nuts, fish, chicken); zinc (oysters, pumpkin seeds, lentils); and iron (red meat, green leaves, kidney beans). Include a daily source of these nutrients in your diet to prevent deficiency.

Did you know?... Some academics have suggested that the reason why Europe remained backward for so long compared to the Middle East was due to widespread iodine deficiency. Arab pioneers wrote about the intellectually challenged Europeans, something which changed when the salt trade opened up around the world.

Noonie Zand Goodarzi

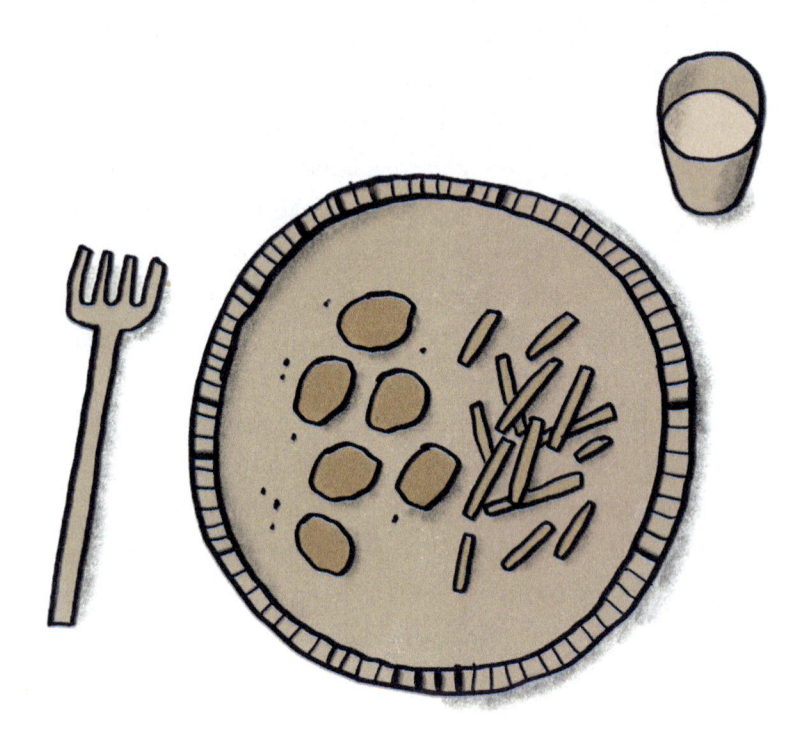

Remember variety is the spice of life

Our bodies were not designed to eat the same thing day after day, week after week. Instead, we would have evolved foraging different plants and occasional meat or fish, all seasonal and highly varied.

Rotating foods has been shown to be a key aspect of good health. Not only do you get more nutrients from a varied diet, but it also increases the diversity of beneficial gut bacteria, essential for immunity, digestion and detoxification. One study of 59,000 women found that those who rotated 16 to 17 healthy foods had a 42 per cent lower mortality from all causes compared to those eating zero to eight healthy foods. What is more, variety was proven even more important than cutting down on unhealthy foods.

Add new ingredients to your shopping list by trying a new recipe every week; get inspiration from shopping at markets; switch up your salads; vary the types of protein, dairy sources (plant and animal) and grains that you eat. Above all, beware a beige-coloured plate and, if you've eaten the same thing three days in a row, move on.

Did you know?... Food intolerances are often a result of a lack of variety. You can develop intolerances from cutting out certain foods for too long *as well as* from over-consuming foods – all the more reason for diversity.

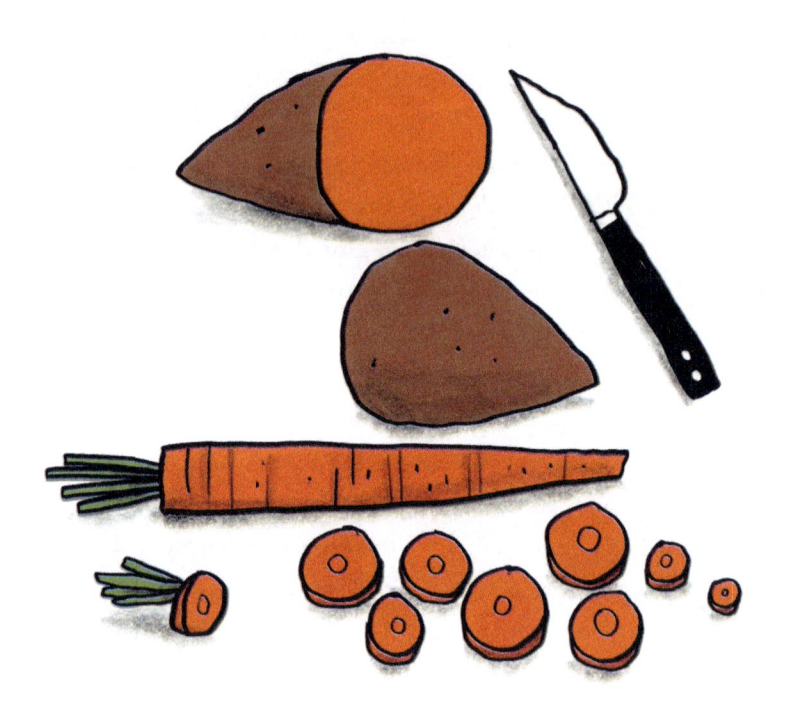

Get rootsy

Root vegetables like sweet potatoes and carrots are some of the healthiest, cheapest and nutrient-dense foods we can buy.

Sweet potatoes are high in fibre and are lower on the glycemic index than white potatoes, which means they have a less immediate impact on blood sugar levels. They are also full of beta-carotene (which converts in the body to vitamin A), which is invaluable for immunity, ageing skin and declining eyesight.

Carrots are pretty impressive too. They contain the antioxidant luteolin which can reduce the brain damage and inflammation seen in dementia. Cooking carrots gives you over six times more vitamin A than raw ones, and cooking them with a little oil boosts absorption even more. Likewise, sweet potatoes with their skins have ten times more antioxidants than the flesh alone.

Try mashed carrots and sweet potatoes instead of normal mash, or mix them in with white potatoes to lower the glycemic load. Include them both when roasting veg, and to soups, or to muffins for a healthy treat.

Did you know?... Christopher Columbus introduced the sweet potato to Europe in the 15th century. The English upper classes revered it for its supposed aphrodisiac properties, which Henry VIII took full advantage of in excessive helpings of spiced sweet potato pie.

Noonie Zand Goodarzi

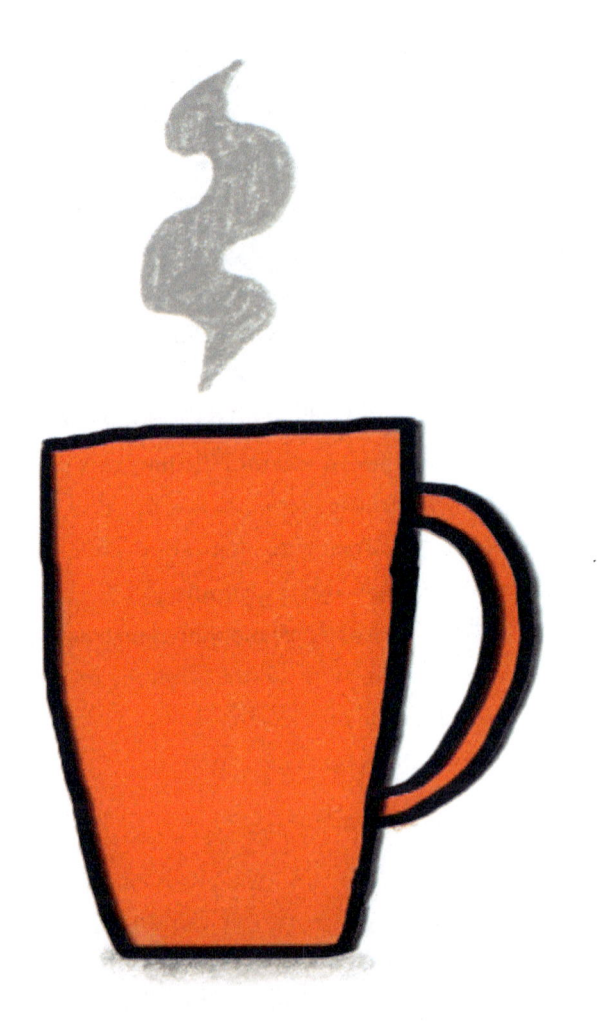

Know your non-dairy milks

Dairy intolerance, veganism and environmental concern has led to a boom in plant-based milks, plus a lot of chatter about their pros and cons. Certainly, not all of them are as healthy as they profess, so if you find yourself using these milks daily, here's the nutritional low down.

Common alternative milks include soya, oat and almond. Soy milk is a good swap for cow's as it contains similar amounts of protein, plus low saturated fat. If you are concerned about its oestrogenic effects, a review of studies on soya found no adverse effects on oestrogen levels in women, or testosterone or oestrogen levels in men.

Oat milk tastes creamy, but it's low in protein, often contains highly processed rapeseed oil, as well as a sugar called maltose that spikes your blood glucose.

Almond milk is low in fat, but also low in protein, and the quantity of almonds in it is typically low – around 2%. Also, almonds and oats are sprayed with harmful pesticides, so organic is best. Watch out for flavours, stabilisers, emulsifiers, thickening agents, preservatives and added sugar.

Did you know?... Plant milks do not contain calcium, iodine or vitamins D and B12 found in cow's dairy, so they are often fortified with them. Organic plant milks cannot be fortified due to certification regulations, so if you go organic, these nutrients must be found elsewhere in the diet.

112   Noonie Zand Goodarzi

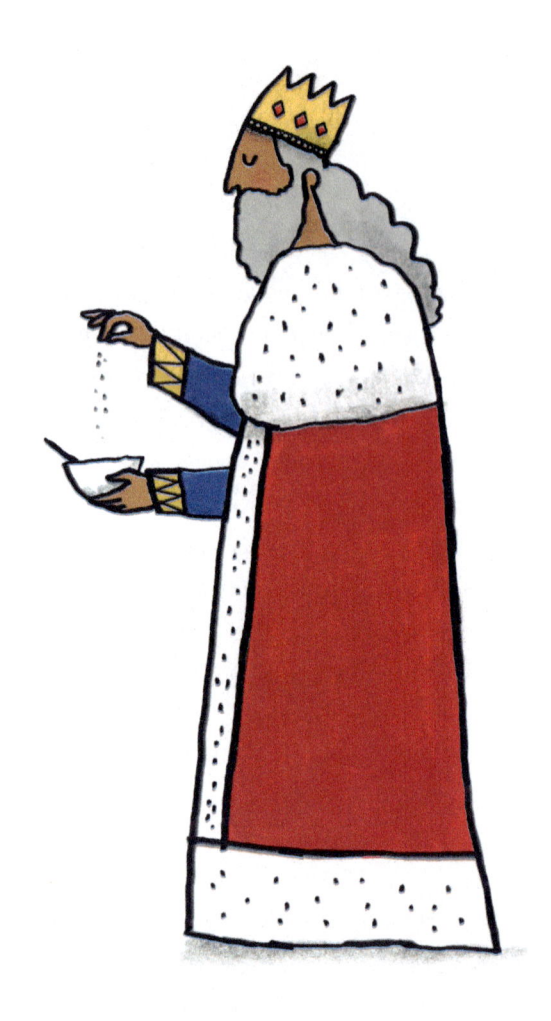

Choose the right cinnamon

Cinnamon is one of those best-beloved spices that takes pride of place in every kitchen spice rack. Its comforting sweet, woody flavour is a friend to puddings and pies, but its health benefits are what really set it apart.

A magic compound called cinnamaldehyde in cinnamon not only helps lower blood sugar (making it good for people with diabetes), but also it has powerful antioxidant activity and has been shown to inhibit the buildup of amyloid-beta plaques, a key sign of Alzheimer's.

Watch out for what type of cinnamon you are using, though. Cassia cinnamon is the more common, cheaper variety, and it contains a compound called coumarin – longterm use of which can be toxic to the liver at doses as little as a teaspoon per day for adults, less for children. Ceylon cinnamon does not contain coumarin, so make the effort to search it out if you like using this spice. Sprinkle on porridge, baked apples, or pears, and try traditional chai tea or golden milk.

> **Did you know?...** For centuries, the origins of cinnamon (the dried bark of a species of laurel tree) were unknown. Traders deliberately kept the route from Ceylon hidden, spinning myths about a perilous journey to faraway lands. This secrecy made cinnamon one of the most coveted commodities in the ancient world, fit for gods and kings.

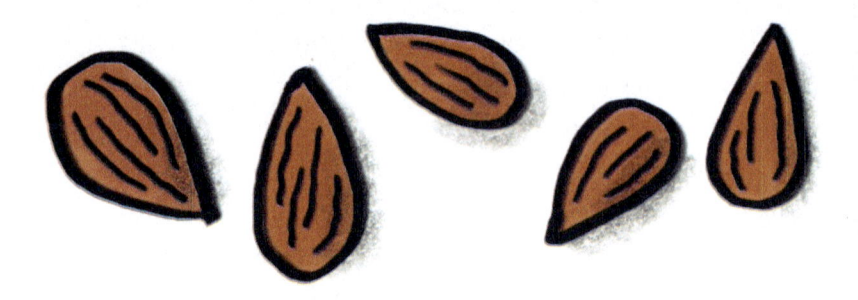

Balance your protein

The current dietary obsession with protein has created the idea that the more protein we eat the better, but this is not entirely true.

Yes, protein plays an important role in weight management; and yes, it is fundamental for muscles and bones, and for making hormones, enzymes and immune cells, but more than the average daily requirement of around 45-55g is unnecessary for good health (unless you exercise a lot). In fact, some long-term population studies have linked high protein intake to greater risk of diseases like heart failure, though the definition of high protein is often problematically vague.

We should still eat protein with every meal as it helps maintain blood sugar balance and increases satiety, but be careful of "protein enhanced" foods like bars and powders which are often ultra-processed. Eat more plant proteins (legumes) than animal protein (red meat), and remember that most plant sources – (except quinoa, soya beans and buckwheat, which *do*) – don't contain all the essential amino acids, or building blocks of protein, that are found in animal protein. To create a complete plant protein, have beans, lentils or chickpeas with brown rice.

Did you know?... 1 medium egg contains 6 grams of protein; small chicken breast = 30g; 1 cup of beans =12g; 1 cup of lentils =18g; a bowl of Greek yoghurt = 20g; milk in regular caffe latte = 8g; handful of almonds = 6g.

Noonie Zand Goodarzi

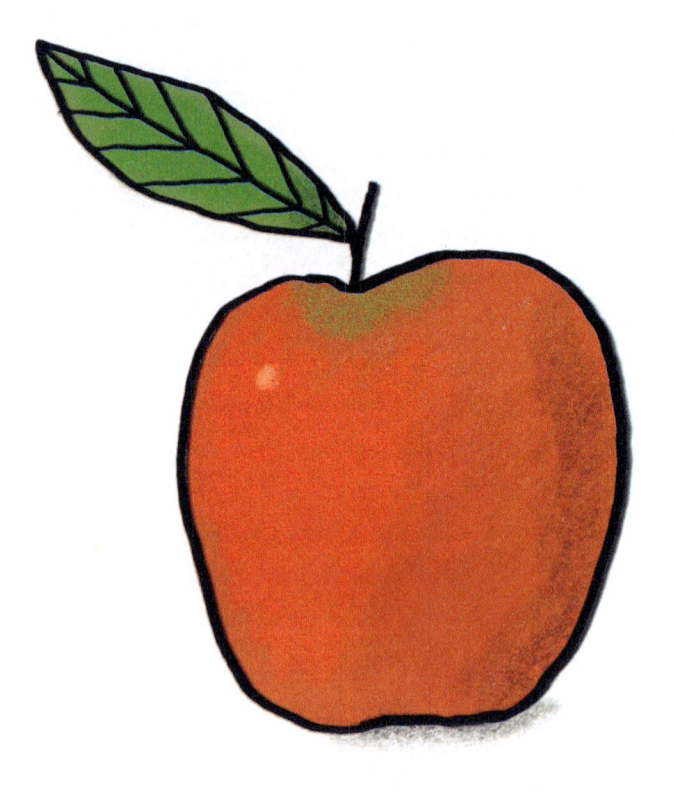

To snack or not to snack?

The inclination to snack throughout the day is a relatively new phenomenon that has been pushed by the food marketing industry. My parents and grandparents never snacked, but nowadays we are persuaded that indulgent treats, mood boosters or comfort foods are what we need.

The science behind the idea that we should eat little and often has changed though, and fasting between meals is now seen as a healthier option. If we eat every couple of hours, our insulin levels never drop and our bodies never use our fat stores for energy. The timing and quality of snacks is also key. The late-night sofa session is one to avoid as the worst time to snack is after 9pm as it causes metabolic turmoil for hours.

Quality snacking means avoiding anything processed, packeted or full of sugar, salt or bad fats – a handful of nuts and seeds, a spoonful of bio-yoghurt with berries, some chopped raw veg with hummus is optimal. People snack the most when at home between 3pm and 8pm, so keep your cupboards free of unhealthy temptations and eat your supper earlier.

Did you know?... Worldwide revenue for snacks and confectionary was a whopping $251.10 billion (US dollars) in 2024. The United States spends $52 billion on snacks every year, followed by China with $27.21 billion and, at the other end of the spectrum, Kenya with $0.7 billion.

Noonie Zand Goodarzi

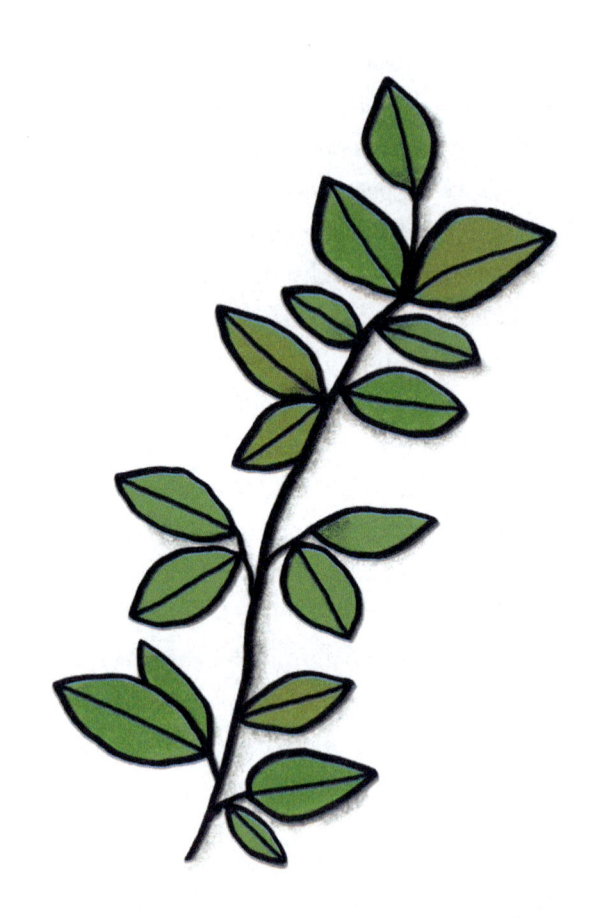

Get a better night's sleep

Everyone knows the horror of lying awake at night, counting down the hours to a difficult day ahead. Sleep is important for a multitude of reasons which makes insomnia all the more stressful. In terms of food, there are lots of do's and don'ts regarding sleep.

DO: try Tart Cherry juice before bed which is high in sleep-inducing melatonin; have an evening cup of turmeric golden milk with a little honey. Milk contains tryptophan which is converted into melatonin and the carbs from the honey help it happen; try valerian and passionflower herb teas which increase levels of calming chemical, GABA; eat dinner at least 4 hours before bed.

DON'T: mindlessly drink caffeine all afternoon; eat high-sugar foods close to bedtime; have spicy food at night as it raises core body temperature which is bad for sleep; drink excess alcohol in the evening as this suppresses the excitatory neurotransmitter glutamate, which might send you off to sleep, but it won't be for long. When the alcohol is fully metabolised in the middle of the night, glutamate levels rebound causing you to wake up and then sleep fitfully.

> **Did you know?...** Electromagnetic radiation from mobile phones and wi-fi routers can interfere with the sleep hormone melatonin's production, as can the blue light emitted from screens. Turn off your mobile and any wi-fi routers within five metres at night to see if this improves sleep.

Acknowledgements

I'd like to thank Niall Edworthy for his boundless encouragement and for overseeing the publication of this book; Mudd Bexley for her brilliant illustrations; and designers Rebecca and Andrew Brown at Principal Publishing.

About the Author

Noonie Zand Goodarzi qualified as a Nutritional Therapist in 2010 at the Institute for Optimum Nutrition (ION), also training at BCNH College of Nutrition and Health and Greenwich University. She has her own practice in Wiltshire, and works as the in-house Nutritional Therapist at a holistic retreat where she gives talks about nutrition and health. Noonie previously worked as a journalist for *The Week* magazine for over 10 years and has an MA (Hons) in English Literature from Edinburgh University.

Printed in Great Britain
by Amazon